Workbook for Mosby's Textbook for the Home Care Aide

3rd edition

Joan Birchenall, RN, MEd
Trenton, New Jersey

Eileen Streight, RN, BSN
Hamilton, New Jersey

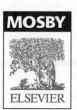

MOSBY

ELSEVIER

ELSEVIER
MOSBY

3251 Riverport Lane
St. Louis, Missouri 63043

WORKBOOK FOR MOSBY'S TEXTBOOK FOR THE HOME CARE AIDE,   ISBN: 978-0-323-08439
THIRD EDITION

Notices

Knowledge and best practice in this field are constantly changing. As new research and experience
broaden our understanding, changes in research methods, professional practices, or medical treatment may
become necessary.

Practitioners and researchers must always rely on their own experience and knowledge in evaluating
and using any information, methods, compounds, or experiments described herein. In using such
information or methods they should be mindful of their own safety and the safety of others, including
parties for whom they have a professional responsibility.

With respect to any drug or pharmaceutical products identified, readers are advised to check the most
current information provided (i) on procedures featured or (ii) by the manufacturer of each product to be
administered, to verify the recommended dose or formula, the method and duration of administration, and
contraindications. It is the responsibility of practitioners, relying on their own experience and knowledge
of their patients, to make diagnoses, to determine dosages and the best treatment for each individual
patient, and to take all appropriate safety precautions.

To the fullest extent of the law, neither the Publisher nor the authors, contributors, or editors, assume
any liability for any injury and/or damage to persons or property as a matter of products liability,
negligence or otherwise, or from any use or operation of any methods, products, instructions, or ideas
contained in the material herein.

Previous editions copyrighted 2003, 1997.

ISBN: 978-0-323-08439-0

Content Strategist: Nancy O'Brien
Senior Content Development Specialist: Maria Broeker
Publishing Services Manager: Deborah L. Vogel
Project Manager: Pat Costigan
Designer: Paula Catalano

Printed in The United States of America

Last digit is the print number: 9 8 7 6 5 4 3 2 1

To the Student

HOW TO USE THIS WORKBOOK

This workbook is designed to help you gain the knowledge and skills needed to begin your career as a home care aide. All of the answers can be found in the corresponding chapters of Mosby's Textbook for the Home Care Aide, third edition. Each set of exercises will help you meet the chapter objectives stated in the text.

Suggestions for using the workbook successfully include:
- Read and follow directions
- Complete each assignment
- Ask your instructor for help if you have any questions or need assistance
- Use the textbook to look up answers that you don't know
- Check your answers with the correct answers provided in this workbook

This workbook gives you the opportunity to be involved in the learning process and to test yourself to see what you have learned and what you still need to study.

Contents

Learning About Home Care

MATCHING

Directions: Match each term listed in Column A with its correct definition in Column B.

Column A

A. Ethnic

B. Client

C. Evaluation

D. Entry-level

E. Certification

F. Confidential

G. Role

H. Clinical experience

Column B

1. ___The usual function of a person

2. ___The process of judging performance to determine progress in learning

3. ___Beginning, just starting

4. ___Practicing skills learned in the classroom in a client care setting

5. ___Person receiving care at home

6. ___Recognition by a government or nongovernment agency that a person has met certain requirements

7. ___A group of people with the same origins or common traits

8. ___Private information that is not to be discussed

SITUATIONS

Directions: Listed below are three situations that involve the home care aide training program. How would you respond to each? Discuss your answers in class.

Situation 1

Your friends are happy that you are starting a new career. They ask you to tell them all about your training program. In the space below, write what you would tell them about your home care training program.

Response:

Length of course _____

Clinical experience _____

Evaluation _____

Situation 2

Before you go to bed, you set out all the things you will need to take to class the next day. Your roommate wants to know why you are taking all these things (notebook, pen, pencils, and textbook) to class.

Response:

_____

_____

Situation 3

Your instructor uses some words that you do not understand. After class, your classmates complain that they don't know the meaning of those "big words" either.

Response:

_____

_____

PRACTICING TO TAKE TESTS

Directions: The following test questions give you a chance to sharpen your test-taking skills. Read each statement carefully, and then give the correct answer. Check your answer at the back of the book to see if you were right or wrong. Good luck!

Examples

True or False

Directions: In the space provided, mark the statement "T" for true or "F" for false. If the statement is false, change it to make it true.

1. ___All home care aide training programs are the same number of hours in length.

2. ___The word *client* refers to a person who is receiving home care.

3. ___The PQRST method is a good way to study.

4. ___The process of evaluating the home care aide's performance only occurs at the end of the program.

5. ___The instructor is the only person who evaluates the student's ability to successfully work in the client's home.

6. ___The ability of the home care aide to work cooperatively with classmates is an important part of being a successful student.

Multiple Choice

Directions: Read carefully and select the best answer for each question. Circle the letter indicating the correct answer. There is only **one** correct answer for each question.

1. Clinical experience takes place:
   a. in the classroom.
   b. in the client's home.
   c. in your own home.
   d. wherever you are learning.

2. When reading the chapter in the textbook, a person should begin with:
   a. stories about clients.
   b. key terms.
   c. chapter objectives.
   d. study questions.

3. Written tests are an example of:
   a. classroom evaluation.
   b. clinical evaluation.
   c. your role.
   d. certification.

REAL-LIFE SITUATIONS

1. How many ethnic groups are represented in your class? Talk to two of your classmates who have a background different from you. Complete the following information:

	Student #1	**Student #2**
Country where the student (or family) was born	_____	_____
Special food they enjoy	_____	_____
Special events	_____	_____
Special customs	_____	_____
Languages they speak/understand	_____	_____

2. Plan a weekly schedule that shows the time you will spend studying or preparing assignments for class. Explain your plan to the people with whom you live, and ask for their support.

2 | The Home Care Industry

MATCHING

Directions: Match each term listed in Column A with its correct definition in Column B.

Column A

A. Official agency

B. Medicaid

C. Chronic illness

D. Hospital discharge planner

E. Assess

F. Diagnostic-related group (DRG)

G. Hospice

H. Reimbursement

I. Acute illness

J. Medicare

K. Standard

L. Policy, policies

M. Voluntary agency

Column B

1. ____A listing of diagnoses used to establish reimbursement by Medicare and Medicaid for hospitalization and medical care

2. ____A federal program of hospitalization, prescription drugs, and health care insurance for persons older than 65 years and/or those with permanent disabilities

3. ____A state and federal insurance program that pays for hospitalization and health care for low-income persons of all ages

4. ____An illness with a rapid onset, severe symptoms, and of short length

5. ____A disease showing little change, slow progress, and of long length

6. ____A program of care that assists the dying client to maintain a satisfactory lifestyle during the end stage of an illness

7. ____A person who arranges for the care of a patient upon release from the hospital

8. ____A gauge that is used as a basis for judgement

9. ____To make payment for an expense incurred

10. ____To determine the client's needs for home care services

11. ____A set of rules and regulations

12. ____An agency sponsored by local or state government

13. ____A nonprofit agency financed through tax-deductible contributions

HIDDEN WORDS: QUALITIES OF A HOME CARE AIDE

Directions: Use the word list below to find the hidden words in the puzzle on p. 5 that describe the qualities of a home care aide. The words may appear from the top down or the bottom up; they may go across, backward, or crosswise. When you find a word, circle it, and then cross off that word in the list.

alert	confident	enthusiastic	patient	skillful
caring	considerate	honest	pleasant	willing
cheerful	cooperative	kind	reliable	
clean	courteous	neat	respectful	
competent	dependable	observant	sincere	

C	E	V	I	T	A	R	E	P	O	O	C	E	P
O	O	E	T	R	E	L	A	P	R	I	O	N	L
M	P	N	L	O	W	I	L	T	T	L	U	T	E
P	A	R	S	B	G	E	N	S	S	U	T	S	A
E	T	L	T	I	A	E	A	C	E	F	N	U	S
T	I	A	B	S	D	I	H	C	N	T	A	O	L
E	E	E	A	I	S	E	L	L	O	C	V	E	U
N	N	N	F	U	E	R	R	E	H	E	R	T	F
T	T	N	H	R	A	K	L	A	R	P	E	R	L
L	O	T	F	E	S	D	I	N	T	S	S	U	L
C	N	U	W	I	L	L	I	N	G	E	B	O	I
E	L	B	A	D	N	E	P	E	D	R	O	C	K
S	I	N	C	E	R	E	G	N	I	R	A	C	S

WORD COMPLETION

Directions: Name the team members who perform the following functions:

Function	Team Member
1. Teaches the client helpful ways to improve swallowing	S _ _ _ _ _-L_ _ _ _ _ _ _
	T_ _ _ _ _ _ _ _
2. Coordinates the activities of the team	C _ _ _ M _ _ _ _ _ _ _
3. Supervises the activities of the LPN/LVN and the home care aide	R _ _ _ _ _ _ _ _ _ _
	N _ _ _ _ _
4. Gives spiritual guidance to the client	C _ _ _ _ _ _
5. Instructs the client and family about preparing meals according to the diet ordered by the doctor	D _ _ _ _ _ _ _ _ _
6. Checks the breathing equipment being used by the client	R _ _ _ _ _ _ _ _ _ _ _ _
	T_ _ _ _ _ _ _ _
7. Arranges community services to be provided to the client	S _ _ _ _ _ _ W _ _ _ _ _ _
8. Provides complex nursing care to clients with special needs	N _ _ _ _ S _ _ _ _ _ _ _ _ _
9. Gives personal care to clients and performs light housekeeping duties	H _ _ _ C _ _ _ _ A _ _ _ _
10. Assesses the client's ability to perform ADL	O _ _ _ _ _ _ _ _ _ _ _ _ _
	T _ _ _ _ _ _ _ _ _ _

11. Gives nursing care to clients whose conditions are stable   L _ _ _ _ _ _ _

                                                             P _ _ _ _ _ _ _ _

                                                             N _ _ _ _ _

12. Teaches exercises to strengthen leg muscles   P _ _ _ _ _ _ _

                                                             T _ _ _ _ _ _ _

TRUE OR FALSE

Directions: In the space provided, mark the statement "T" for true or "F" for false. If the statement is false, change it to make it true.

1. ___The needs of the client and family determine the kinds of members required on the home care team.

2. ___You develop an earache while you're at work. You may take your client's prescription drug, provided you request permission.

3. ___The registered nurse is responsible for evaluating the progress of the therapy given to the client by the physical therapist.

4. ___When visitors arrive, sit down and talk with them.

5. ___It is the case manager's job to assess the kinds of services required by each client.

6. ___An example of client services provided by a community agency is home-delivered meals.

7. ___It is not necessary to maintain healthy eating habits if you provide good client care.

8. ___First impressions are usually lasting ones.

9. ___Your client's husband is drinking beer while he's eating lunch and offers you one, too. It's okay to have one beer, but not more.

10. ___The client's family asks you to work extra hours for which they will pay you. This is acceptable, provided that they do not notify the agency of this arrangement.

3 Developing Effective Communication Skills

TRUE OR FALSE

Directions: In the space provided, mark the statement "T" for true or "F" for false. If the statement is false, change it to make it true.

1. ___Hearing-impaired persons will understand what you are saying if you exaggerate your words.

2. ___It is helpful to keep a pad and pencil nearby so that your visually-impaired client can communicate in writing, if necessary.

3. ___Speak to the side where the client's hearing is better.

4. ___Turn off the television and household appliances to reduce background noise before speaking to a hearing-impaired client.

5. ___Touching a visually-impaired client's hand to get and keep attention is a good idea.

6. ___Always stand to the side of visually-impaired clients, because their side vision is good.

7. ___If possible, turn off exposed light bulbs and lower window shades to reduce glaring light when talking to a client who has poor vision.

8. ___Speak in a loud tone of voice to make sure that your blind client understands what you are saying.

9. ___While your client, Mr. Jackson, is asking you a question, be sure to concentrate on how you will answer him.

10. ___You know the answer to the question Maria Gonzales is asking, but you wait until she is finished talking before you respond.

11. ___The client has the right to refuse treatment.

12. ___The client has the right to refuse care given by an African-American home care aide.

13. ___Your client, who looks sad, is wearing heavy makeup that exaggerates her lips and eyebrows in an unbecoming way. You should compliment her on how attractive she looks to make her feel better.

14. ___The client has the right to know the plan of care in advance.

15. ___The home care aide has the right to be treated with respect and dignity by the client and family.

SITUATIONS

Directions: Listed below are three situations you may experience as a home care aide. How would you respond? What would you do? Discuss your answers with your classmates.

Situation 1

You have been caring for your client, Sarah Walker, for several months. Her husband, Ben, has always been very friendly, and he compliments you on your appearance and the quality of care that you provide each time you visit.

During your last visit, Ben asked you to go into the bedroom while Sarah was eating her breakfast in the kitchen. He said he wanted to talk about his wife's illness. When the two of you were in the bedroom, he said, "I just want to talk to you alone. You are very special to me. I think you like me, too." Then, he reached for your hand.

Response:

_____

_____

Action:

_____

_____

Situation 2

This is your first day with a new client, Joseph D'Orio, who is 87 years old and very confused. He lives with his son, his daughter-in-law, and two adult grandchildren.

While giving Mr. D'Orio a bath, you notice several bruises on his back and burn marks on his arms and legs. You ask Joseph about them, and he starts to cry. He says that his son doesn't love him anymore because he is such a burden.

Response:

_____

_____

Action:

_____

_____

Situation 3

You have been making daily visits to care for Amy Doyle, a disabled child who is 3 years old. Each day for the last week, Amy's mother has been telling you how hard it is for her to pay for the rent, gas, electricity, and food.

Today, you arrive on the job, and there is no heat or electricity in the apartment. Amy's mother asks you to call the gas company to have the services restored.

Response:

_____

_____

Action:

_____

_____

Situation 4

As you are putting on your coat to leave your client's apartment, her son Harry says, "You have been very kind to my mother for these past 6 months, and I really appreciate all that you have done for her. I just wanted you to have this. I know that it's not much, but we all can use some more cash during the holidays." Then, he tries to put some folded five-dollar bills into your hand.

Response:

_____

_____

Action:

_____

_____

MATCHING

Directions: Match each term listed in Column A with its correct definition in Column B.

<table>
<tr>
<td>Column A</td>
<td>Column B</td>
</tr>
<tr>
<td>A. Communication</td>
<td>1. ___One who is appointed to act for another</td>
</tr>
<tr>
<td>B. Verbal communication</td>
<td>2. ___A wrong, considered grounds for a formal complaint</td>
</tr>
<tr>
<td>C. Nonverbal communication</td>
<td>3. ___Sharing of thoughts, information, and opinions with others</td>
</tr>
<tr>
<td>D. Bias(es)</td>
<td>4. ___To like or dislike someone or something without a good reason</td>
</tr>
<tr>
<td>E. Prejudice</td>
<td>5. ___Communication using the spoken or written word</td>
</tr>
<tr>
<td>F. Disability</td>
<td>6. ___Code of behavior or conduct</td>
</tr>
<tr>
<td>G. Surrogate</td>
<td>7. ___Physical, mental, or emotional condition that interferes with activities of daily living</td>
</tr>
<tr>
<td>H. Advance directive</td>
<td>8. ___Something spoken or written in confidence, in secret</td>
</tr>
<tr>
<td>I. Grievance</td>
<td>9. ___Communication without the use of words</td>
</tr>
<tr>
<td>J. Confidentiality</td>
<td>10. ___Document that indicates a client's wishes about health care</td>
</tr>
<tr>
<td>K. Ethics</td>
<td>11. ___Having or forming a preconceived judgement or opinion without fair reasons</td>
</tr>
</table>

DIAGRAM

Directions: Label the diagram (Figure 3-1) using the terms listed below.

Message   Meaning   Sender   Receiver   Feedback

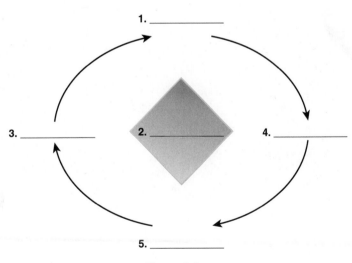

1. _____

2. _____

3. _____

4. _____

5. _____

Figure 3-1

COMPLETION

Directions: Fill in the blanks to complete each sentence.

1. Effective communication begins with one basic principle: _____

   _____.

2. Five ways to improve listening skills are:

   a. _____;

   b. _____;

   c. _____;

   d. _____;

   e. _____.

3. Two topics to avoid when communicating with your client are _____

   and _____.

4. Confidential information is shared with your supervisor when _____

   _____.

5. To be a good listener, you must devote _____
   to the speaker.

4 Understanding Your Client's Needs

DIAGRAM

Directions: Label the pyramid (Figure 4-1) to show the basic human needs as described by Maslow. Use the words listed below, and write in the appropriate space.

Love   Physical   Self-actualization   Security and safety   Self-esteem

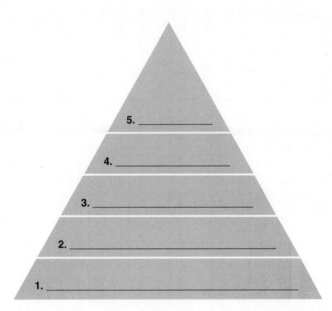

5. _____

4. _____

3. _____

2. _____

1. _____

Figure 4-1

COMPLETION

Directions: Complete the following statements.

1. Oxygen and food are examples of _____ needs.

2. Preventing falls helps to meet a client's need for _____.

3. Feeling close to other persons helps to meet the need for _____.

4. Feeling good about oneself is meeting the need for _____.

5. By learning and creating, people meet their need for _____.

TRUE OR FALSE

Directions: In the space provided, mark the statement "T" for true or "F" for false. If the statement is false, change it to make it true.

1. ___We all belong to a nuclear family.

2. ___The word *family* always refers to one's mother, father, and siblings.

3. ___There is no typical family.

4. ___Many families are mobile—moving from place to place.

5. ___The most important structure in society is the family.

6. ___Family members always work together to meet all of their own needs.

7. ___The home care aide meets all of the needs of the client and family.

8. ___The needs of the client come first.

9. ___Home care aides have no personal needs.

10. ___When needs are unmet, physical and emotional problems can arise.

GROWTH AND DEVELOPMENT

Directions: List five principles of growth and development:

1. _____

2. _____

3. _____

4. _____

5. _____

GROWTH AND DEVELOPMENT CHART

Directions: Complete the chart below.

Development Stage	Age	Characteristics	Ways to Meet Client Needs
Infancy		1. Tremendous growth	1. Hold and cuddle
	to 1 year	2.	2.
		3.	3.
Toddler	1–3 years	1. Endless activity	1. Eliminate hazards
		2.	2.
		3.	3.
Preschool	____ years	1. Endless energy	1. Avoid use of "don't"
		2.	2.
		3.	3.
School age	6–12 years	1.	1.
		2.	2.
		3.	3.
Adolescent	____ years	1.	1.
		2.	2.
		3.	3.
Adulthood	18–65 years	1.	1.
		2.	2.
		3.	3.
Older adulthood	65–100+ years	1.	1.
		2.	2.
		3.	3.

5 Understanding How the Body Works

IDENTIFICATION

Directions: In the space provided, identify the body system that contains the listed organ.

Organ	System
1. Pituitary gland	_____
2. Liver	_____
3. Prostate gland	_____
4. Bronchioles	_____
5. Diaphragm	_____
6. Ribs	_____
7. Arteries	_____
8. Gallbladder	_____
9. Capillaries	_____
10. Ovaries	_____
11. Urethra	_____
12. Spinal cord	_____
13. Larynx	_____
14. Brain	_____

FILL IN THE BLANKS

Directions: For each body system, give the appropriate function.

Body System	Function
1. Skeletal	_____
2. Muscular	_____
3. Circulatory and lymphatic	_____
4. Integumentary	_____
5. Nervous	_____
6. Respiratory	_____
7. Endocrine	_____
8. Digestive	_____
9. Urinary	_____
10. Reproductive	_____

MATCHING

Directions: Match each definition listed in Column A with the correct term in Column B.

Column A	Column B
A. Basic functioning unit of the body	1. ___Villi
B. Blood cells are produced here	2. ___Nephron
C. The exchange of oxygen and carbon dioxide takes place here	3. ___Small intestine
D. Basic functioning unit of the kidney	4. ___Nerves
E. Digestion of food is completed here	5. ___Hormones
F. Stores urine	6. ___Large intestine
G. Secretions that enter the bloodstream from glands	7. ___Alveoli
H. Sends messages to other parts of the body	8. ___Long bones
I. The structure that sends food into the bloodstream	9. ___Bladder
J. Absorbs fluid back into the body	10. ___Cell

COMPLETION

Directions: Fill in the blanks to complete each sentence.

1. Tissues are made up of groups of _____.

2. Another word for *throat* is _____.

3. Arteries carry blood _____ the heart.

4. _____ connect arteries to veins.

5. A heart beat has two parts: _____ and _____.

6. A body system is made up of many _____.

7. Another word for *windpipe* is _____.

8. The lid that prevents food from entering the respiratory system is the _____.

9. The long, strong muscles are in the _____.

10. The urethra has two functions in the man because it carries both _____ and _____.

DIAGRAM

Directions: Fill in the blanks next to each figure (Figures 5-1, 5-2, and 5-3).

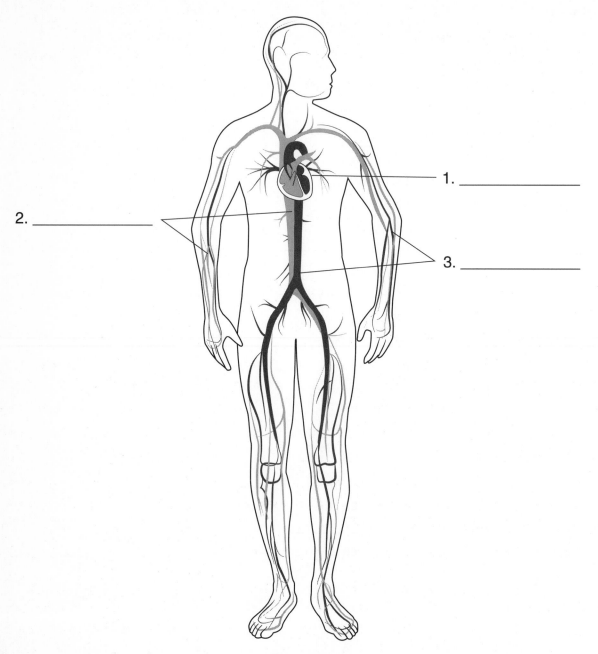

1. _____

2. _____

3. _____

Figure 5-1

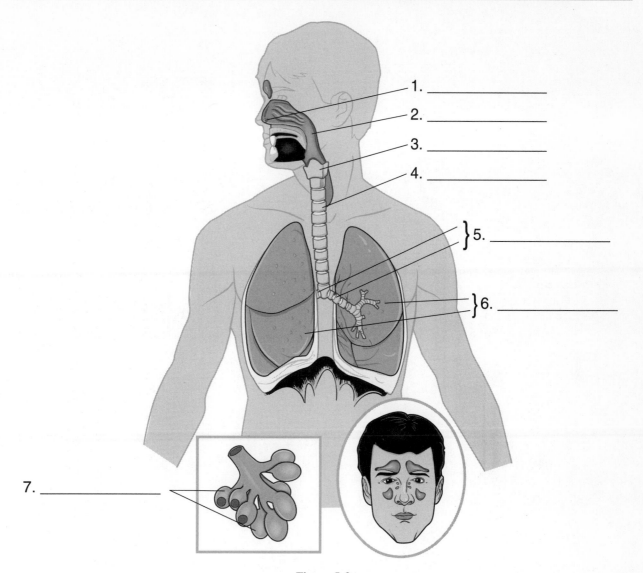

1. _____
2. _____
3. _____
4. _____
5. _____
6. _____
7. _____

Figure 5-2

2. _____

1. _____

3. _____

7. _____

4. _____

8. _____

9. _____

5. _____

10. _____

6. _____

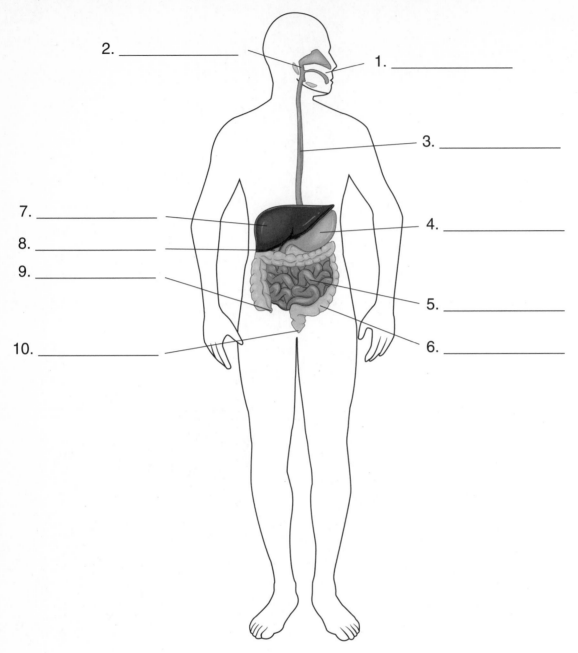

Figure 5-3

6 Observing, Reporting, and Recording

MATCHING

Directions: Match each prefix, suffix, or root word listed in Column A with its correct definition in Column B.

Column A	Column B
A. -itis	1. ___Blood
B. gastro-	2. ___New opening
C. arthr-	3. ___Pain
D. -uria	4. ___Stomach
E. -stomy	5. ___Inflammation
F. cerebr-	6. ___Surgical removal
G. hyper-	7. ___Under
H. post-	8. ___Urine or urination
I. -ectomy	9. ___Cerebrum
J. hem-	10. ___Joint
K. hypo-	11. ___Above
L. -algia	12. ___After

REPORTING AND RECORDING

Directions: Next to each observation, indicate the action that you would take to report and record the information.

1. Bruise on client's arm _____

2. Client complains of sudden pain in chest _____

3. Foul odor in client's refrigerator _____

4. Client having severe difficulty with breathing _____

5. Client has sudden vomiting and diarrhea _____

6. Client's toilet overflowed; client lives alone and has no immediate family nearby _____

7. Client refused lunch and drank one cup of tea _____

8. Client cried for half an hour after brother's visit _____

9. Client's daughter slapped client twice in the face during a 15-minute visit _____

10. Client had been irritable but now is pleasant and talkative _____

TRUE OR FALSE

Directions: In the space provided, mark the statement "T" for true or "F" for false. If the statement is false, change it to make it true.

1. ___Client care records are permanent, written, legal documents.

2. ___The care record can be shared with family members.

3. ___The entire care record is kept in the client's home.

4. ___Home care aides usually chart on a checklist.

5. ___Client care records may be used as evidence in court cases.

6. ___Always use a pen when writing on a client record.

7. ___Change the care plan if you believe that this is necessary.

8. ___The vital signs are the temperature, pulse, respirations, and blood pressure.

9. ___The agency should be notified whenever you observe changes in the client's physical or mental condition.

10. ___You shouldn't call your supervisor too much; you don't want to be a pest.

ABBREVIATIONS

Directions: Give the meanings of the following abbreviations:

1. abd   _____

2. ADL   _____

3. BP   _____

4. CA   _____

5. meds   _____

6. O_2 _____

7. OOB   _____

8. ROM   _____

9. Tbsp   _____

10. TPR   _____

11. c̄   _____

12. mL   _____

13. s̄   _____

14. tsp   _____

RECORDING

Directions: Complete the Weekly Client Care Record—Change in Condition section of Figure 6-1 on p. 23 for the following scenario:

Ten minutes after you arrive at your client's home (9:10 AM), she vomits her breakfast. She complains of feeling dizzy, her skin is bluish, and her breathing is noisy. You call 9-1-1, your supervisor, and your client's sister, who is upstairs. Your client is taken to the medical center by the ambulance at 9:45 AM, and her sister goes with her. Your supervisor comes to the client's home.

WEEKLY CLIENT CARE RECORD

Client _____   Employee _____

Address _____   Title _____

City _____ State _____ Zip _____   Client or Account # _____

Phone (day) _____ (eve.) _____   Week Ending _____ / _____ / _____

Fill in the date for each day.

Write your initials in the box which corresponds to each task performed.

	DATE							
	DAY	Mon.	Tue.	Wed.	Th.	Fri.	Sat.	Sun.
	TIME ARRIVED							

PERSONAL CARE:

	Mon.	Tue.	Wed.	Th.	Fri.	Sat.	Sun.
Bath ☐ Bed ☐ Chair ☐ Shower ☐ Tub							
Perineal Care							
Hair ☐ Groom ☐ Shampoo							
Mouthcare ☐ Denture Care							
Shave							
Nail Care ☐ Clean ☐ File							
Foot Care							
Special Skin Care							
Dressing ☐ Assist ☐ Complete							
Toileting ☐ Bed Pan ☐ Commode ☐ BRP							
Other instructions: _____							

CLIENT ACTIVITIES:
Transfer Activity Instructions: _____

	Mon.	Tue.	Wed.	Th.	Fri.	Sat.	Sun.
Assist with walking ☐ Cane ☐ Walker ☐ Crutches							
Assist with exercises ☐ ROM ☐ Other (specify)							
Wheelchair activities							
Other instructions: _____							

OTHER FUNCTIONS:

	Mon.	Tue.	Wed.	Th.	Fri.	Sat.	Sun.
Temp. ☐ Oral ☐ Rectal ☐ Underarm ☐ Ear							
Pulse							
Respirations							
Blood Pressure							
Weigh Client							
Record Intake/Output (use special form)							

Figure 6-1

Continued

	Mon.	Tue.	Wed.	Th.	Fri.	Sat.	Sun.
OTHER FUNCTIONS:							
Prepare and serve meal/snack							
Special diet (Specify)							
Assist with feeding							
Medications reminder							
Stoma care							
Incontinent care							
Record bowel movements							
Change in condition (office was notified)							
Other instructions: _____							
HOUSEHOLD SERVICES:							
Change/make client's bed							
Clean client's room							
Clean bathroom							
Clean kitchen; wash dishes							
Vacuum, sweep, dust							
Client laundry							
Marketing							
Errands (specify) _____							
Other instructions: _____							
DEPARTURE TIME							
TOTAL HOURS							

I certify that the hours shown represent my true total hours worked.

Signature _____   Title _____   Date _____

Return form to Home Care Agency weekly.
Notify Home Care Agency if your client's condition has changed since your last visit.

Figure 6-1, cont'd

WEEKLY CLIENT CARE RECORD—CHANGE IN CONDITION

Date	Time	Observation	Action Taken

Signed: _____

Figure 6-1, cont'd

CHECKLIST

Directions: Complete the Weekly Client Care Record (Figure 6-1) for the following:

Client OOB to chair
Wash, dry, and fold client's personal laundry and linens
Assist client with shower and dressing
Clean client's bathroom
Change and make client's bed
Weigh client daily before shower

SITUATION

Directions: Fill in the blanks about the following situation:

Your client, Mr. Leo, tells you that he has "indigestion." He says, "It must be from the fried eggs and sausage that I had for breakfast." He asks you to get his "indigestion medicine."

List three actions that you should take:

1. _____
2. _____
3. _____

INCIDENT REPORT

Directions: Complete an incident report (Figure 6-2, p. 24) for the following situation:

When you step onto the porch at your client's home, your left foot goes through a weak board. You fall, scrape your left leg, and hurt your left ankle, which becomes swollen and painful. You limp into the client's home and call your supervisor. He comes over to assess your injury, takes you to the emergency department for treatment, and completes an incident report.

ABC Home Care Agency
INCIDENT REPORT

PERSON INVOLVED	(Last name)	(First name)	(Middle initial)

Address _____   Adult ☐   Child ☐   Male ☐   Female ☐   Age _____

Date of incident/accident	Time of incident/accident A.M. ☐ P.M. ☐	Exact location of incident/accident

Bedroom ☐   Hallway ☐   Bathroom ☐   Other ☐ Specify _____

CLIENT ☐   List diagnosis if contributed to incident/accident:

Client's condition before incident/accident

Normal ☐   Confused ☐   Disoriented ☐   Sedated ☐ (Drug_____ Dose _____ Time _____)   Other ☐ Specify _____

Were bed rails ordered? Yes ☐ No ☐	Were bed rails present? Yes ☐ No ☐	If Yes, Up ☐ Down ☐	Was height of bed adjustable? Yes ☐ No ☐	If Yes, Up ☐ Down ☐

EMPLOYEE ☐   Name _____   Job title _____   Length of time in this position _____

VISITOR ☐   OTHER ☐   Home address _____   Home phone _____

Occupation _____   Reason for presence _____

Equipment involved ☐
Property involved ☐   Describe _____   Was person authorized to be at location of incident/accident? Yes ☐ No ☐

Describe exactly what happened; why it happened; what the causes were. If injury, state part of body injured. If property ot equipment damaged, describe damage.

_____
_____

Indicate on diagram location of injury:

Temp. _____   Pulse. _____   Resp. _____

B.P. _____

TYPE OF INJURY

1. Laceration   ☐
2. Hematoma   ☐
3. Abrasion   ☐
4. Burn   ☐
5. Swelling   ☐
6. None apparent   ☐
7. Other (specify below)   ☐
_____

LEVEL OF CONSCIOUSNESS
_____
_____

Name of supervisor notified	Time of notification _____ A.M./P.M.	Time of responded _____ A.M./P.M.
Name and relationship of family member notified	Time of notification _____ A.M./P.M.	Time of responded _____ A.M./P.M.

Was person involved seen by a physician? Yes ☐ No ☐ If Yes, physician's name	Where	Date	Time	A.M. ☐ P.M. ☐
Was first aid administered? Yes ☐ No ☐ If Yes, type of provided by whom	Where	Date	Time	A.M. ☐ P.M. ☐
Was person involved taken to a hospital? Yes ☐ No ☐ If Yes, hospital name	By whom	Date	Time	A.M. ☐ P.M. ☐

Name, title (if applicable), address & phone no. of witness(es)	Additional comments and/or steps taken to prevent recurrence:

SIGNATURE/TITLE/DATE	**SIGNATURE/TITLE/DATE**
Person preparing report	Case Manager
Supervisor	Administrator

INCIDENT REPORT

Figure 6-2 (Modified from Briggs Corporation, Des Moines, Iowa.)

7 Working With Ill and Disabled Clients

CLIENT REACTIONS

Directions: Read the following client situations. In the space provided, identify the client's reaction, and explain what you would do.

1. Hector, who is able to feed himself, has finished half of his meal. You observe that he has had difficulty controlling his fork today. Therefore, you suggest that he use a spoon to finish eating his food. Suddenly, Hector takes the fork and throws it across the room.

   A. Hector is demonstrating _____.
   B. What would you do?

   _____

   _____

   _____

2. You enter Rita's bedroom to begin preparing for her bed bath. She does not respond to your greeting, and she turns her back toward you as you speak to her.

   A. What is Rita's reaction called? _____
   B. What would you do?

   _____

   _____

   _____

3. Maria has weak leg muscles, and the physical therapist has instructed her to perform exercises each day. When you ask her to show you the exercises, she says, "I really don't think I can do them. What will happen if I fall? I'm so weak." Then she wrings her hands and shakes her head "No."

   A. Maria's response shows _____.
   B. What would you do?

   _____

   _____

   _____

4. Sam is being cared for by his wife, who says that she does "everything" for him. Your supervisor has given you instructions to encourage Sam to perform his own activities of daily living (ADL). When you give Sam a washcloth to clean his face, he says, "You wash me. My wife always does it for me."

   A. Sam is demonstrating _____.
   B. What would you do?

   _____

   _____

   _____

5. Robert has diabetes and is on a severe sugar-restricted diet. You prepare his lunch according to the food require-ments ordered by the doctor. Robert says that the food you prepare is "okay" but that he "likes lots of sweets." His daughter tells you that he hides candy in his bedroom and eats it when he's watching television at night. When he is asked why he eats all that candy, Robert says, "It won't hurt me. I know the doctor made a mistake. I'm not a diabetic."

A. Robert's response shows _____.
B. What would you do?

_____

_____

_____

FAMILY SITUATIONS

Directions: Read the following family situations. In the space provided, answer the question asked about each situation.

1. Mrs. Tucker tells you that she feels like everything she does for her husband is "all wrong." He is nasty, he com-plains, and he wants things right away. Mr. Tucker has been ill for the past 5 years, and he is becoming increasingly unable to perform ADL. His wife says, "I am so tired, so hurt, and so disgusted! I just don't know what to do. I could sit here and cry all day." As the home care aide, what could you do to help the Tucker family?

_____

_____

2. Ann Marie Burroughs is a 17-year-old high school student who was diagnosed with cancer of the bone. Her leg was amputated above the knee. After the surgery, she is at home waiting for her artificial limb to be delivered and fitted. Meanwhile, she is crutch walking using the remaining limb. You are helping Ann Marie with her personal care at home, including bathing, grooming, and other ADL. Ann Marie spends most of her day crying. She will not see any of her friends, she does not answer the telephone, and she refuses to work with the home teacher. Ann Marie says her life is over, that she might as well be dead, and that she is never going back to school or out of the house again. Her mother is very concerned and asks you what can be done to help her daughter.

_____

_____

3. Jose Santiago, who is 36 years old, has to care for both of his parents, who are 72 years old. Jose's father has had a stroke; he is paralyzed on one side of the body and is unable to care for himself. Jose's mother fell and fractured her hip. She uses a walker, and she needs assistance with personal care and grooming. Jose is doing all of the housekeeping, shopping, and cooking. He says that he has no income during this period and that things are really getting tough. His parents' Social Security checks don't seem to go far enough, and the rent, utility bills, car payment, and auto insurance are all due. Jose tells you that he is very anxious because he needs to work, yet his parents need his help and care, too. What would you do to help the Santiago family?

_____

_____

_____

CROSSWORD PUZZLE

Directions: Complete the crossword puzzle by identifying the important terms found in Chapter 7.

Across

1. Avoids contact with others
4. Prolonged feeling of intense sadness
6. Duties and responsibilities assumed by a person
7. Refusal to admit the truth
8. Loss of ability to perform certain functions
10. State of relying too much on others

Down

2. Feeling very mad
3. State of physical, mental, and social well-being
5. Absence of health
9. State of intense worry and/or fear

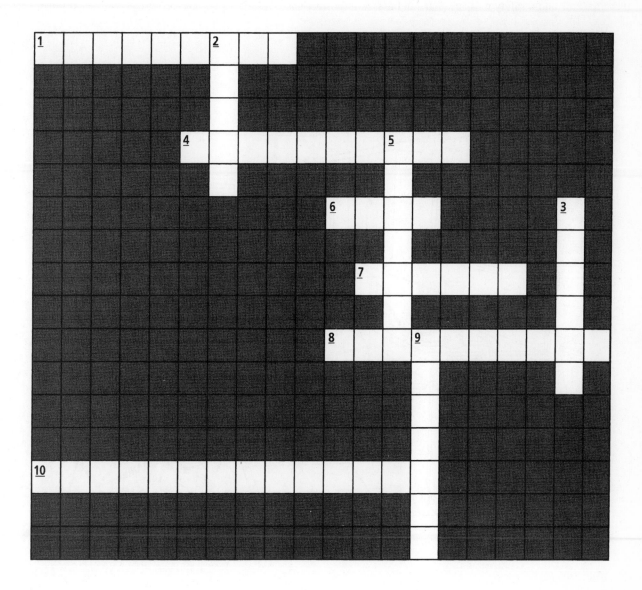

8 | Maintaining a Safe Environment

HOME HAZARDS

Directions: In the picture below (Figure 8-1), there are more than 10 safety hazards. In the space provided, list 10 of these hazards and a safety measure that can be used to correct each.

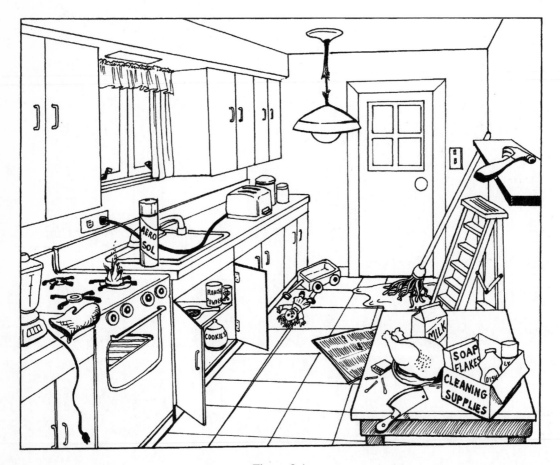

Figure 8-1

Hazards

1. _____
2. _____
3. _____
4. _____
5. _____
6. _____
7. _____
8. _____
9. _____
10. _____

Safety Measures

1. _____
2. _____
3. _____
4. _____
5. _____
6. _____
7. _____
8. _____
9. _____
10. _____

DIAGRAM

Directions: Label the diagram below (Figure 8-2) to show the three ingredients that combine to start a fire. Give two examples of each ingredient.

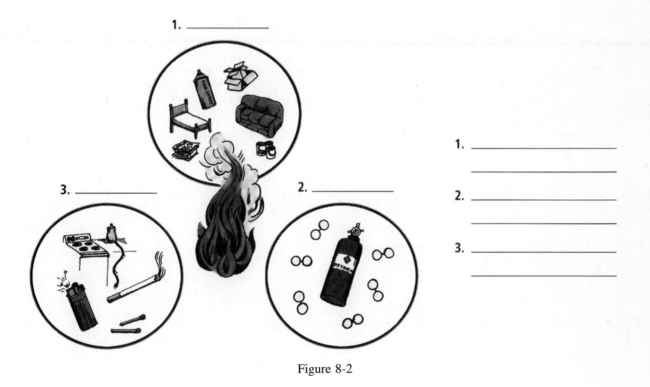

Figure 8-2

MATCHING

Directions: Match each item listed in Column A with one of the ingredients needed to start a fire listed in Column B.

Column A

1. ___Cigarettes

2. ___Pilot light

3. ___Clothing

4. ___Air

5. ___Cigarette lighter

6. ___Medical oxygen

7. ___Elevator shaft

8. ___Pot holders

9. ___Open doors leading to fire exits

10. ___Frayed electrical cord

11. ___Oily rags

12. ___Stacks of old newspapers

Column B

A. Fuel

B. Oxygen

C. Heat source

SITUATIONS

Directions: Fill in the blanks about the following situations:

1. Willie Mae Jones takes the bus to get to and from her client's eighth-floor apartment in the city. The bus stop is two blocks from her home. She then walks three more blocks to reach her client's apartment house. This area has many small stores that are open for business during the day but that are closed when she waits for the 6 PM bus to go home.

   A. List three personal safety rules that Willie Mae should remember when walking to and from the bus stop and waiting for the bus.

      1. _____

      2. _____

      3. _____

   B. List three safety rules to remember when riding the bus.

      1. _____

      2. _____

      3. _____

   C. List three safety precautions that Willie Mae needs to take before reaching the door of her client's apartment or her own home.

      1. _____

      2. _____

      3. _____

2. Ethel's client lives on a farm. Ethel uses her own car to travel the 20 miles from her home to the farmhouse. There are no gas stations on this route; there is one roadside restaurant and only two houses, which are located a half mile off of the road. Ethel is concerned about her safety while traveling this rural road, especially after dark. List eight safety rules that you would encourage Ethel to remember while traveling to and from her client's home.

1. _____

2. _____

3. _____

4. _____

5. _____

6. _____

7. _____

8. _____

3. You have been asked to gather ideas for a disaster supply kit. Of the items listed below, select those you would use when preparing the kit by writing "Yes" or "No" in the space provided.

_____Blanket

_____Eating utensils

_____Pots and pans

_____Money, including coins

_____First aid kit

_____Extra car keys

_____Flashlight, including batteries

_____Important papers (e.g., insurance policies, wills)

_____Essential medications in childproof containers

_____Sweater

_____Canned food and can opener

_____Bottle of liquor

_____Bottle of water

_____Shampoo

_____Hairspray

9 Maintaining a Healthy Environment

HOUSEHOLD TASKS SCHEDULE

Directions: In the space next to each household task, write whether the task should be performed weekly or daily.

Making the client's bed _____

Cleaning the refrigerator _____

Cleaning the commode _____

Changing the bed linens _____

Removing trash _____

Laundering bed linens _____

Picking up clutter _____

Washing dishes _____

Dusting the living room _____

Cleaning the toilet and the bathroom sink _____

Sweeping the kitchen floor _____

Cleaning the kitchen counters _____

CLEANING AND STORING SUPPLIES

Directions: Describe how each of the following items should be cared for after use.

Dust cloth _____

Broom _____

Sponge _____

Bucket _____

Toilet brush _____

Rubber utility gloves _____

SORTING LAUNDRY

Directions: The items of clothing listed in the left column below need to be sorted into appropriate washer loads. For each item, select the type of load to which it belongs.

____1. Dirty work clothes

____2. White cotton athletic socks

____3. Blue toilet lid cover

____4. Cotton print dress

____5. Nylon underwear

____6. White cotton sheets

____7. Blue jeans

____8. Light purple towels

____9. Dark brown cotton tee shirt

____10. Yellow jogging top and pants

____11. Diapers

____12. Pink embroidered sweater

A. Sturdy white

B. Dark

C. Colorfast

D. Heavily soiled

E. Delicate

TRUE OR FALSE

Directions: In the space provided, mark the statement "T" for true or "F" for false. If the statement is false, change it to make it true.

1. ____Sick people are not able to care for their own homes.

2. ____The client's physical needs come before housekeeping duties.

3. ____Always work from the cleanest to the dirtiest area.

4. ____Use a bag or basket to collect clutter.

5. ____Use a sharp knife to remove frost from a freezer.

6. ____Wash wooden bowls in the automatic dishwasher.

7. ____Use baking soda solution to clean the refrigerator.

8. ____When treating linens that are stained with body fluids, wear gloves.

9. ____Never mix chlorine bleach with ammonia.

10. ____Do not make comments about your client's poor housekeeping.

11. ____Wear protective gloves when using household cleaning solutions.

12. ____Read garment care labels before washing clothes.

10 Meeting the Client's Nutritional Needs

FILL IN THE BLANKS

Directions: Fill in the blanks to complete each sentence.

1. Food energy is measured by means of a unit called a _____.

2. Carbohydrates are composed of the chemicals _____, _____, and _____.

3. Sugars and starches are examples of _____.

4. Amino acids are components of _____.

5. Vitamins A, D, E, and K are _____-_____vitamins.

6. A tool to use during menu planning is the_____ _____ _____.

7. The five groups of the MyPlate Food Guide are _____, _____, _____, _____, and _____.

8. Too much saturated fat may increase the level of _____ in the blood.

9. *Roughage* is another word for _____.

10. The term that is used to describe poor appetite is _____.

11. When assisting a blind client to eat, the plate is described as a _____.

12. Foods that are high in salt are avoided on a _____-restricted diet.

13. Spicy, highly seasoned, and fried foods are avoided when following a _____diet.

14. The human body is _____ percent fluid.

15. The daily need for water (fluids) is at least _____.

16. A lack of fluid in the body can cause _____.

17. Three factors to consider during menu planning are_____, _____, and _____.

18. Butter, cream, and ice cream would be avoided on a _____-_____ diet.

19. Proper storage is essential to preserve the _____ and _____of foods.

20. Calcium and phosphorus are examples of _____ found in food and needed by the human body.

CROSSWORD PUZZLE

Directions: Complete the crossword puzzle by identifying the important terms found in Chapter 10.

Across

1. Microorganisms that cause disease

3. Food needed for body growth and repair

4. Having excessive water loss from body tissues

6. Process by which food is taken in and used by the body

Down

2. Disorder of nutrition

5. Lack of one or more nutrients in the diet

7. Method of pricing food

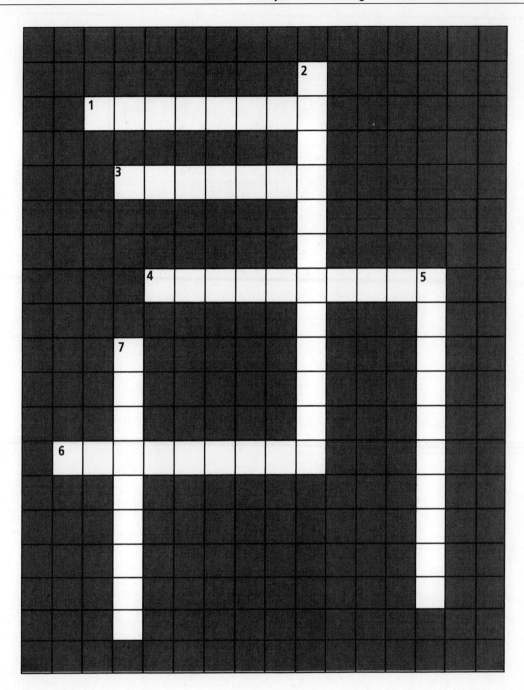

MYPLATE FOOD GUIDE

Directions:
1. Identify each food group of the MyPlate Food Guide (Figure 10-1).

A. _____

B. _____

C. _____

D. _____

E. _____

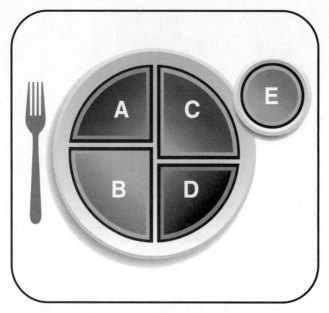

Figure 10-1

2. Name three foods that are included in each food group shown in Figure 10-1.

A. _____

_____

_____

B. _____

_____

_____

C. _____

_____

_____

D. _____

_____

_____

E. _____

_____

_____

MATCHING

Directions: Match the eating problems listed in Column A with the different ways to prepare clients' meals listed in Column B. There may be more than one correct match for each item in Column B.

Column A

A. Low energy levels

B. Difficulty chewing

C. Difficulty swallowing

D. Poor appetite

Column B

1. ___Avoid serving crackers.

2. ___Prepare attractive, colorful meals.

3. ___Use drinking straws.

4. ___Avoid celery stalks and raw carrots.

5. ___Serve thick, soft foods.

6. ___Cut food into small pieces.

7. ___Use thickeners in fluids.

8. ___Use lightweight cups and glassware.

9. ___Serve fluids about 1 hour before meals.

10. ___Cut meat and butter bread.

11. ___Prepare small meals and snacks.

12. ___Add gelatin to cold liquids.

13. ___Allow plenty of time for eating.

THERAPEUTIC DIETS

Directions: Change the regular diet menu in Column A to meet the requirements of the diets listed in Columns B, C, and D (Figure 10-2).

A REGULAR	B SOFT	C SODIUM RESTRICTED	D LOW FAT
Canned or Homemade Soup			
Ham Sandwich on Bread			
Mayonnaise			
Lettuce and Tomato			
Whole Milk			
Cookies			

Figure 10-2

SITUATIONS

Directions: Listed below are three situations you may experience as a home care aide. In the space provided, supply the missing information.

1. Your client has prepared the following shopping list. Indicate next to each item the additional information that you will need from the client before you go shopping.

   Milk _____

   Bread _____

   Orange juice _____

   Eggs _____

   Ground beef _____

   Carrots _____

   Bananas _____

   Broccoli _____

   Toilet tissue _____

   Ice cream _____

2. When you return from purchasing the items on the shopping list, they must be stored properly. Where will you store them to preserve quality and maintain freshness?

   Milk _____

   Bread _____

   Orange juice _____

   Eggs _____

   Ground beef _____

   Carrots _____

   Bananas _____

   Broccoli _____

   Toilet tissue _____

   Ice cream _____

3. Your client, Mrs. Smith, tells you that she wants to go to the new food warehouse to see whether the prices there are cheaper than those at the supermarket. She tells you to put her wheelchair in the back of your car and drive her there. What is your response? What would you do?

   Response: _____

   Action: _____

11 Preventing Infection/Medical Asepsis

MATCHING

Directions: Match each term listed in Column A with its correct definition in Column B.

Column A	Column B
A. Standard (universal) precautions	1. ___Free from all living organisms
B. Pathogenic	2. ___Specialized clothing or equipment worn by an employee for protection against a biohazard
C. Disinfection	3. ___Process that destroys pathogenic organisms
D. Host	4. ___Occurs when harmful organisms enter the body and grow, causing illness and disease
E. Carrier	
F. Sterile	5. ___Rules to follow to prevent bloodborne disease
G. Personal protective equipment	6. ___A person or animal in which microorganisms live
H. Exposure incident	7. ___Pathogenic microorganisms that are present in human blood and can cause disease in humans
I. Bloodborne pathogen	
J. Medical asepsis	8. ___Usually not capable of causing or producing a disease
K. Infection	9. ___Capable of causing a disease
L. Nonpathogenic	10. ___Situation when client's blood may enter the health care worker's body
	11. ___A person or animal that spreads disease to others but does not become ill
	12. ___Use of techniques and practices to prevent the spread of pathogenic organisms

TRUE OR FALSE

Directions: In the space provided, mark the statement "T" for true or "F" for false. If the statement is false, change it to make it true.

1. ___Always wear gloves when cleaning up blood spills.

2. ___Standard (universal) precautions should be taken only if your client has Acquired Immunodeficiency Syndrome (AIDS).

3. ___When in doubt about disinfecting certain items in the home, ask the client.

4. ___Wash your hands after removing gloves.

5. ___Microorganisms are only found in the human body.

6. ___An individual's skin acts as a natural defense against infection.

7. ___OSHA regulations concerning bloodborne pathogens must be followed by doctors and nurses only.

8. ___When masks or gowns become wet, they are no longer effective barriers against pathogens.

9. ___Three signs of infection are pain, swelling, and redness of the area.

10. ___Remove rings before applying gloves.

COMPLETION

Directions: Fill in the blanks to complete each sentence.

1. To grow and multiply, all microorganisms need _____, _____, and _____; or _____, _____, and _____.

2. Boil items for _____ minutes to destroy pathogenic organisms.

3. When preparing vinegar solution, use _____ part vinegar to _____ parts water.

4. Disinfection using the oven requires that items be baked for _____ at a temperature of _____° F (_____° C).

5. When preparing bleach solution, use _____ part bleach to _____ parts water.

6. Bleach solution must be put in a plastic container. The label must contain this information: _____, _____, and _____.

7. Handwashing is required _____ and _____ giving client care.

8. The most common household disinfecting solution is _____ or _____ and _____ _____.

9. Microorganisms can be transmitted by means of _____, _____, _____, _____or _____ human contact, _____, and _____.

10. Factors that help to increase the risk for infectious diseases include:

    a. _____

    b. _____

    c. _____

    d. _____

    e. _____

SITUATIONS

Directions: In the space provided, answer the questions asked about each situation.

1. As you remove the linens from your client's bed, you are stuck by an uncapped needle on an insulin syringe that was accidently left in the bed. What would you do?

   _____

   _____

   _____

2. Mr. Werts is coughing up sputum and spitting it into an old coffee can. He wants you to empty the can into the toilet and return it to him. What would you do?

   _____

   _____

   _____

3. Mrs. Hunt uses two disposable insulin syringes each day. She also uses four lancets (i.e., short, pointed blades) to collect blood to test her sugar level. How would Mrs. Hunt safely discard these sharps?

   _____

   _____

4. Your client has had an "accident" in bed. The client, his clothing, and the bed linens are soiled with urine and feces. Describe the following:
   The protective equipment that you would use:

   _____

   _____

   How you would transport the soiled clothing and linen to the laundry area in the basement of the home:

   _____

   _____

   _____

   How you would pretreat and launder the soiled linens:

   _____

   _____

   _____

CYCLE OF INFECTION

Directions: Label the six parts of the cycle of infection in the drawing below (Figure 11-1).

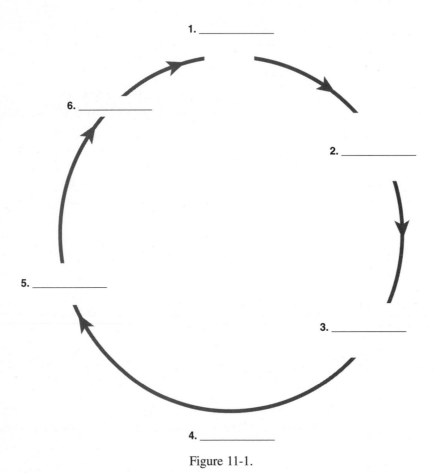

1. _____

2. _____

3. _____

4. _____

5. _____

6. _____

Figure 11-1.

12 Body Mechanics

Body Mechanics

PROCEDURES

Directions: Listed below are five procedures (including six major steps for each) used to assist clients to move in and out of bed. For each procedure, review the steps listed and number them in the correct order.

1. Applying a transfer (gait) belt:

    ___Apply the belt over the client's clothing and around his or her waist.

    ___Place the belt buckles off center in the front or back.

    ___Explain what you are going to do.

    ___Wash your hands.

    ___Assist the client to sit on the side of the bed.

    ___Tighten the belt until it is snug.

2. Standing transfer from bed to chair/wheelchair:

    ___Lock the wheelchair brakes, and place the footrests out of the way.

    ___Wash your hands.

    ___Assist the client to sit at the side of the bed.

    ___Have the client reach back and grasp the farthest armrest of the chair or wheelchair with one hand and then to do the same with the nearest armrest.

    ___Place the wheelchair parallel to the client's bed on the client's strong side.

    ___Place your arms under the client's arms and around the client's back, and lock your fingers together.

3. Assist the client to sit on the side of the bed:

    ___Provide privacy.

    ___Help the client to put on a robe and footwear.

    ___Lock the wheels on the bed or push the bed against the wall if there are no brakes.

    ___Place the client in Fowler's position.

    ___On the count of "3," shift your weight to your back leg, and slowly swing the client's legs over edge of bed while pulling his or her shoulders to a sitting position.

    ___Explain what you are going to do.

4. Raising the client's head and shoulders:

    ___Explain what you are going to do.

    ___Slip your farthest arm under the client's neck and shoulders.

    ___Rock the client to a semisitting position.

    ___Wash your hands.

    ___Lower the head of the bed, and remove pillows.

    ___Lock arms with the client on the side that is nearest to you.

5. Moving the client to the side of the bed:

___Explain what you are going to do.

___Place arms underneath the client.

___Move the client in three segments from the center of the bed to the edge of the bed.

___Stand with your feet apart.

___Shift your weight from your front leg to your back leg when moving the client.

___Wash your hands.

IDENTIFY THE INCORRECT POSTURE

Directions: What is wrong with the following pictures (Figures 12-1, 12-2, and 12-3)? In the space provided, explain how you would correct the picture.

1. Figure 12-1: _____

_____

_____

_____

_____

_____

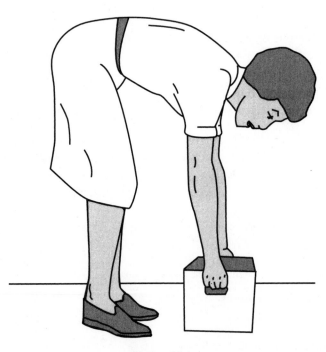

Figure 12-1

2. Figure 12-2: _____

_____

_____

_____

_____

_____

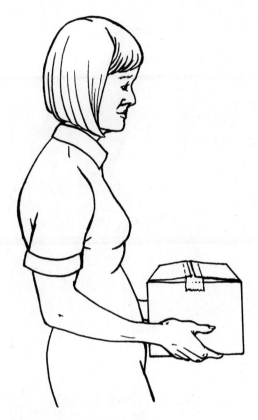

Figure 12-2

3. Figure 12-3: _____

_____

_____

_____

_____

_____

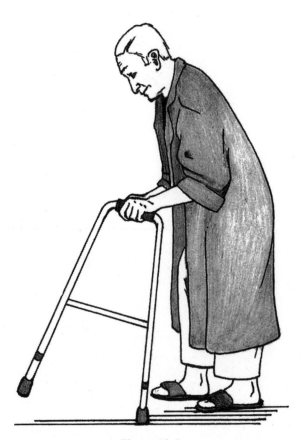

Figure 12-3

MATCHING

Directions: Match each term listed in Column A with its correct definition in Column B.

Column A	Column B
A. Body mechanics	1. ___To walk
B. Shearing	2. ___Example of assistive device
C. Contractures	3. ___Device to keep weight of upper bedding off client's feet and legs
D. Bed cradle	4. ___Loss of ability to move
E. Ambulate	5. ___Pressure against surface of skin and skin layers as client is being moved
F. Pressure ulcer	6. ___Proper use of muscles to move and lift objects
G. Fatigue	7. ___Inflammation of the lung
H. Pneumonia	8. ___Muscles shorten and joints become permanently immovable
I. Walker	9. ___Loss of strength and endurance
J. Immobility	10. ___Sore on the skin caused by prolonged pressure on the part (bed sore)

SITUATIONS

Directions: Read the following situations. In the space provided, answer the question asked about each situation.

1. This is your first visit with Mr. Rand, a 65-year-old man who is recovering from surgery to repair a fractured hip. The physical therapist has been teaching Mr. Rand exercises to strengthen his leg and arm muscles. Mr. Rand's girlfriend usually helps him to get out of bed to practice these exercises. During your visit, you explain to Mr. Rand how he can help you as you assist him with getting out of bed. He responds, "Oh, no, that's not how my girlfriend does it." The girlfriend then tells you how she helps him, and you learn that what she is doing is incorrect and that it is unsafe for both her and Mr. Rand. What would you do?

_____

_____

_____

2. As your client walks from her living room to the kitchen, she complains of dizziness and begins to fall. You ease her to the floor. She complains of feeling faint and weak. What would your next action be?

_____

_____

_____

IDENTIFY THE POSITION

Directions: Write the name of the position next to each figure (Figures 12-4 through 12-8).

1. _____

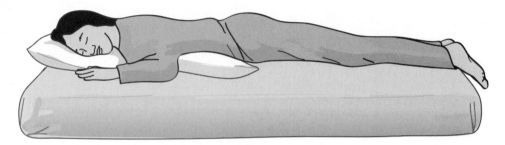

Figure 12-4

2. _____

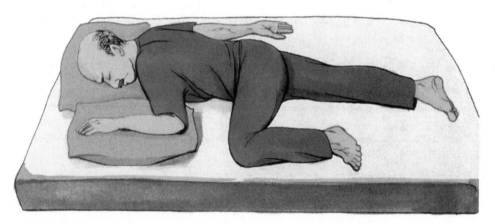

Figure 12-5

3. _____

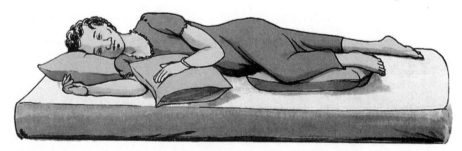

Figure 12-6

4. _____

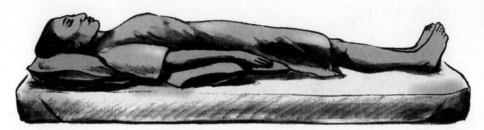

Figure 12-7

5. _____

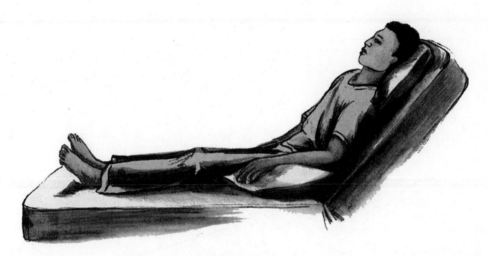

Figure 12-8

SAFETY FACTORS

Directions: List 10 safety factors to consider when positioning, moving, and lifting clients.

1. _____
2. _____
3. _____
4. _____
5. _____
6. _____
7. _____
8. _____
9. _____
10. _____

13 Bedmaking

DIAGRAM

Directions: In the space provided, identify the linens that are used on the bed (Figure 13-1).

A. _____

B. _____

C. _____

D. _____

E. _____

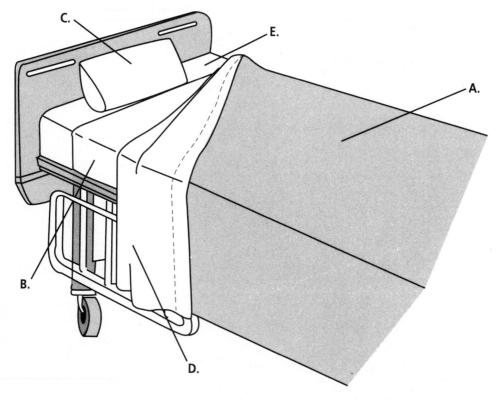

Figure 13-1

TRUE OR FALSE

Directions: In the space provided, mark the statement "T" for true or "F" for false. If the statement is false, change it to make it true.

1. ___Provide privacy for your client before making an occupied bed.

2. ___Always wear gloves when handling linens that have been stained with body fluids.

3. ___The materials that you use to make the bed depend on the client's needs and what is available.

4. ___If the top sheet is not soiled, it may be reused as a bottom sheet.

5. ___Use a dry cleaner's bag if the bed needs a plastic drawsheet.

6. ___A closed bed is made while the client remains in the bed.

7. ___When possible, get your client out of bed before making it.

8. ___Roll soiled linens away from your clothing.

9. ___Shake the bed linens to remove any crumbs.

10. ___Do not place your client directly on a plastic drawsheet.

11. ___Hold soiled linens close to you so that you won't drop them on the floor.

12. ___Fanfold the top bedding to the foot of the bed to open a closed bed.

13. ___A bed cradle is used to lift the top bedding off of the client's feet.

14. ___The most important reason for making a clean, neat, wrinkle-free bed is to make the bed look nice.

15. ___Wash the egg-crate foam mattress pad when it becomes soiled.

14 Personal Care

PROCEDURES

Directions: Listed below are six procedures used to assist clients with personal care and grooming. For each procedure, review the steps that are listed, and then number them in the correct order.

1. Giving a back rub:

   ___Remove excess lotion with a towel.

   ___Place the client on his or her side or abdomen to expose the entire back.

   ___Remove clothing from the client's upper body.

   ___Rub your hands together to warm the lotion.

   ___Use long, firm, but gentle strokes—up, out, and down.

   ___Provide privacy (close door, shut drapes, and pull shades).

2. Giving a complete bed bath:

   ___Wash the client's genital and rectal areas.

   ___Give the client a back rub.

   ___Remove soiled towels and washcloths, and place in an area so that they will be washed.

   ___Wash and dry one of the client's legs while other foot is soaking.

   ___Obtain materials.

   ___Wash the client's eye areas gently with clean water only.

3. Giving a shower in the bathtub:

   ___Adjust water temperature and water pressure.

   ___Assist client into the tub and to use the grab bars.

   ___Clean the tub, and remove the towels to an area to be washed.

   ___Place a nonskid mat in the tub.

   ___Place a bath chair in the tub.

   ___Check the temperature of the bathroom for warmth, and be sure that the room is free of drafts.

4. Shaving a male client with a blade razor:

   ___Explain what you are going to do.

   ___Put on gloves.

   ___Wet and lather the client's face.

   ___Remove the gloves, and wash your hands.

   ___Shave in the direction of hair growth.

   ___Obtain materials.

5. Caring for the client's hair:

___Brush the client's hair, section by section, from the root to the end of the hair.

___Explain what you are going to do.

___Wash your hands.

___Place a bath towel around client's shoulders.

___Remove the towel.

___Arrange the client's hair as client wishes.

6. Caring for the client's dentures:

___Assist the client to remove dentures from mouth.

___Wash your hands, and put on gloves.

___Fill the sink with warm water.

___Assist the client to replace dentures in mouth.

___Brush the dentures with toothpaste and rinse them.

___Obtain materials.

TRUE OR FALSE

Directions: In the space provided, mark the statement "T" for true or "F" for false. If the statement is false, change it to make it true.

1. ___All clients need complete personal care.

2. ___The term *oral hygiene* refers to the care of the mouth, including the teeth, gums, and tongue.

3. ___Dentures are cleaned in hot, soapy water.

4. ___Older adults may take a tub bath or shower twice a week.

5. ___Not everyone needs a daily bath.

6. ___Partial baths may be given in bed, at the bedside, or in the bathroom.

7. ___Any chair may be used in the shower.

8. ___The proper water temperature for a bath or shower is 109°F (42.7°C).

9. ___Electric razors are not used when clients are receiving oxygen, because there is a danger that an electrical spark could cause a fire.

10. ___When helping clients to dress, put clothing on their weak side first.

11. ___With range-of-motion (ROM) exercises, the client lifts weights and performs deep knee bends.

12. ___Stop ROM if you feel resistance or tightness in the client's joint.

13. ___Do as much as you can for your client; this will help him or her to get better faster.

14. ___Always wear gloves when shaving a client's face with a blade razor.

15. ___False teeth should be stored in a denture box or cup.

WHAT NEEDS TO BE CORRECTED?

Directions: In the figures that follow, there are problems with personal care. In the space provided, explain how you would correct the picture.

1. (Figure 14-1)

   A. What's wrong?

   _____

   B. Correction:

   _____

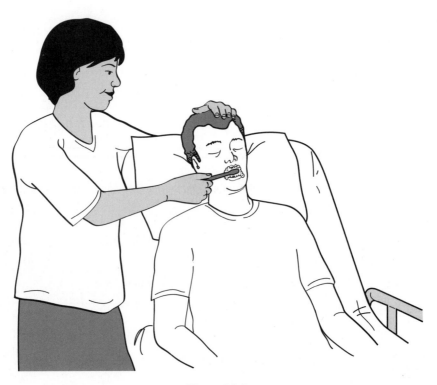

Figure 14-1

2. (Figure 14-2)

   A. What's wrong?

   _____

   B. Correction:

   _____

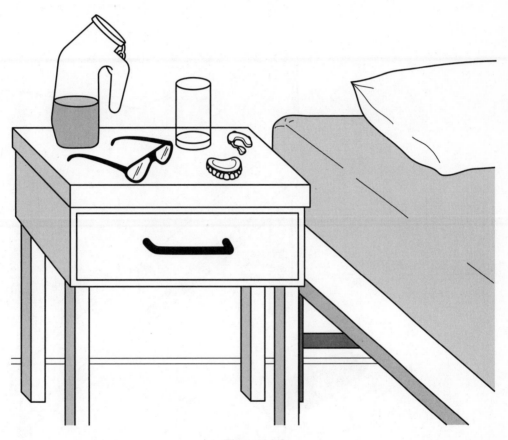

Figure 14-2

3. (Figure 14-3)

   A. What's wrong?

   _____

   B. Correction:

   _____

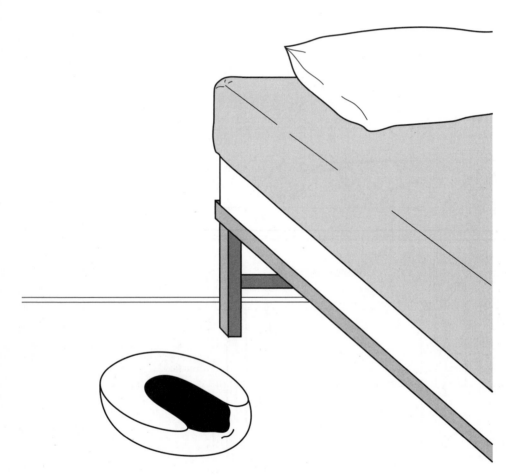

Figure 14-3

4. (Figure 14-4)

  A. What's wrong?

  _____

  B. Correction:

  _____

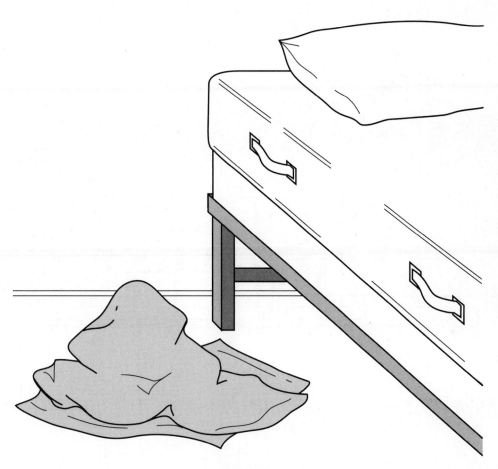

Figure 14-4

5. (Figure 14-5)

   A. What's wrong?

   _____

   B. Correction:

   _____

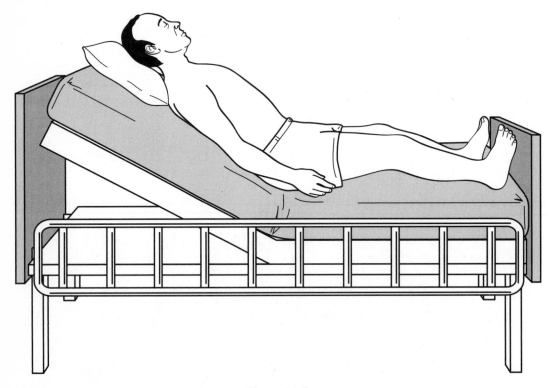

Figure 14-5

15 Elimination

PROCEDURES

Directions: Listed below are four procedures used to assist clients with elimination. For each procedure, review the steps listed, and then number them in the correct order.

1. Giving and removing a bedpan:

   _____Give the client toilet tissue, and ask the client to call you when finished.

   _____Place the client in a flat position, and remove the bedpan.

   _____Raise the bed to a convenient working height.

   _____Cleanse the client's perineal area with toilet tissue, if necessary, wiping from front to back.

   _____Warm the bedpan with warm tap water, and then dry it with paper towels.

   _____Cover the bedpan, take it to the bathroom, and empty its contents.

2. Giving and removing a urinal:

   _____Give the urinal to the client so he can position it properly.

   _____Help the client to wash hands.

   _____Rinse the urinal with cold water, and then clean and disinfect it.

   _____Put on gloves, and remove the urinal.

   _____Assist client to stand.

   _____Put the urinal away, and remove and discard the gloves.

3. Caring for a client with an indwelling catheter:

   _____Record what you have done, and report any abnormal conditions.

   _____Put on gloves.

   _____Tape and position the catheter properly.

   _____Give perineal care.

   _____Remove the waterproof protector pad.

   _____Wash the catheter tube in a downward motion, away from the urinary meatus, for approximately 4 inches (20 cm).

4. Applying a condom catheter:

   _____Put on gloves.

   _____Connect the catheter tip to the drainage tubing.

   _____Give perineal care.

   _____Remove and discard the gloves.

   _____If a condom catheter is present, remove it gently, and place in a plastic bag.

   _____Hold the client's penis firmly, and roll the condom catheter onto the penis, with drainage opening at the urinary meatus.

WHAT NEEDS TO BE CORRECTED?

Directions: In the figures that follows, problems with catheter bags and tubing are shown. In the space provided, explain what you would correct in each picture.

1. (Figure 15-1)

A. What's wrong?

_____

B. Correction:

_____

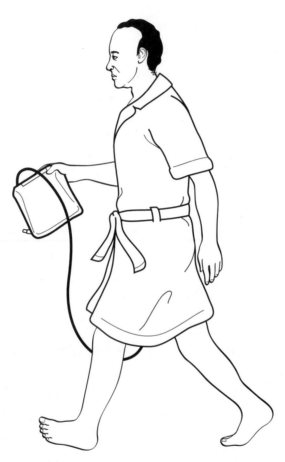

Figure 15-1

2. (Figure 15-2)

   A. What's wrong?

   _____

   B. Correction:

   _____

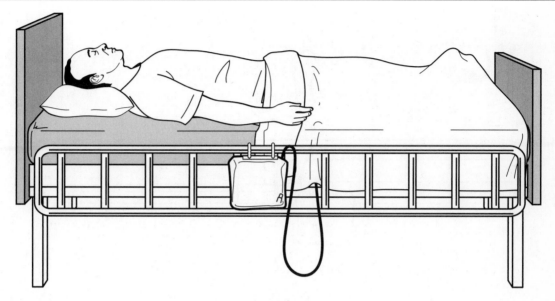

Figure 15-2

3. (Figure 15-3)

   A. What's wrong?

   _____

   B. Correction:

   _____

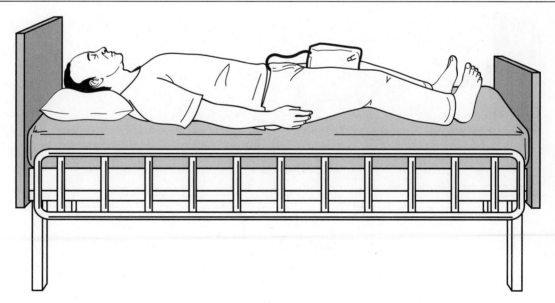

Figure 15-3

4. (Figure 15-4)

   A. What's wrong?

   _____

   B. Correction:

   _____

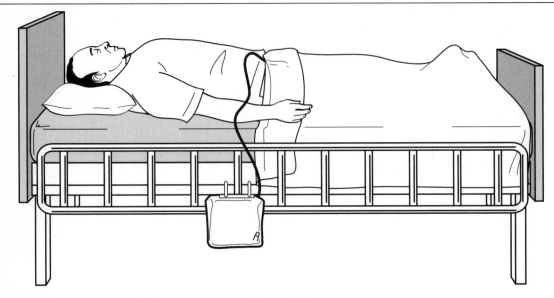

Figure 15-4

5. (Figure 15-5)

   A. What's wrong?

   _____

   B. Correction:

   _____

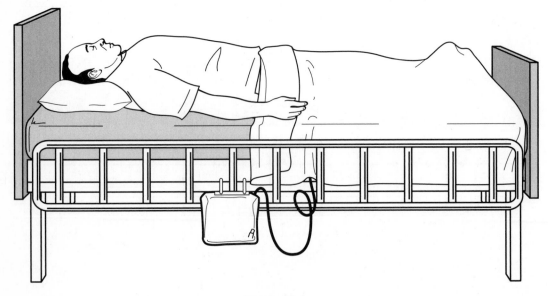

Figure 15-5

SITUATIONS

Directions: In the space provided, answer the questions about each situation.

1. Your client is on I&O. During the 4 hours that you provide care for Mr. Abud, he does the following:
   Voids 375 mL of urine
   Drinks one cup of tea
   Eats two 8-oz cups of gelatin and four crackers
   Has one small bowel movement
   At the end of your 4-hour shift, you record the client's I&O as follows:

   I = _____ mL

   O = _____ mL and _____.

2. Miss O'Brien was in the hospital for 1 week. During that time, she had difficulty with bowel elimination. Now that she is home, the doctor wants her to reestablish her normal bowel habits. Miss O'Brien uses the commode at her bedside. List three things that you can do to help her to regain her regular bowel habits.

   A. _____

   B. _____

   C. _____

3. Your client, Juanita, has an indwelling catheter. While providing her perineal care, you observe that the area around the catheter is leaking urine and that the skin is very reddened. She says that the area is painful and that she always has the feeling of wanting to use the commode. List two actions that you would take to handle this situation.

   A. _____

   B. _____

4. Mr. Patel has a colostomy. He is learning to care for it himself, but he needs help with unclamping and draining the pouch of fecal material. Mr. Patel's companion tells you that Mr. Patel cries a lot after the registered nurse visits to instruct him about caring for the colostomy.
   A. What will you say to Mr. Patel's companion?

   _____

   _____

   _____

   B. List three duties that you may need to perform when helping Mr. Patel with colostomy care.

   (1) _____

   (2) _____

   (3) _____

COMPLETION

Directions: Fill in the blanks to complete each statement.

1. Three characteristics of normal urine are _____, _____, and _____.

2. Two characteristics of a normal bowel movement (BM) are _____ and _____.

3. The medical term that is used to describe air or gas in the intestine that is passed through the rectum is _____.

4. Two kinds of gas-forming foods are _____ and _____.

5. When clients are not able to control urination or bowel movements, the medical term used to describe this condition is _____.

6. If you notice changes in your client's urine or bowel movements, notify your _____.

7. Your client has not had a BM for over 1 week, and he complains of abdominal discomfort. Also, you notice that small amounts of fecal liquid leak out of the client's anus. These may be signs that your client has a

_____.

8. Waste materials are eliminated from the body by _____, _____,

_____, and _____.

9. The medical term for material that is eliminated from the large intestine is _____.

10. The medical term that is used to describe the process of eliminating solid waste through the anus is _____.

11. When waste products in the large intestine move so rapidly that the water is not able to be absorbed, this is called

_____.

12. When providing perineal care or removing a bedpan, it is important to _____.

13. Three ways to help clients to maintain normal urination are:

A. _____

B. _____

C. _____

16 Collecting Specimens

PROCEDURES

Directions: Listed below are three procedures used to collect clients' specimens. For each procedure, review the steps listed, and then number them in the correct order.

1. Collecting a routine urine specimen:

   _____Pour the urine into the graduated cylinder and then into the specimen container until $\frac{3}{4}$ full.

   _____Label the container.

   _____Store the specimen in the refrigerator.

   _____Have the client void into a commode, bedpan, urinal, or "hat."

   _____Put the lid on the specimen container.

   _____Remove and discard gloves.

2. Collecting a stool specimen:

   _____Explain what you are going to do.

   _____Transfer the stool to the specimen container using a tongue depressor.

   _____Label the container.

   _____Put on gloves.

   _____Record what you have done, and report any abnormal conditions to your supervisor.

   _____Flush any remaining feces down the toilet, and help the client to complete toileting as necessary.

3. Collecting a sputum specimen:

   _____Place the container into a plastic bag and then into a paper bag.

   _____Have the client hold the sputum specimen container.

   _____Remove and discard gloves.

   _____Obtain materials.

   _____Do not touch the inside of the container. Keep the outside of the container clean and free of any sputum.

   _____Help the client to rinse mouth with plain water.

TRUE OR FALSE

Directions: In the space provided, mark the statement "T" for true or "F" for false. If the statement is false, change it to make it true.

1. _____Specimens are small amounts of body tissue or fluids that are collected for examination and analysis in the medical laboratory.

2. _____Have the client discard used lancets directly into the garbage can.

3. _____Label specimen container with the client's name and the agency's name.

4. _____Specimen containers are capped tightly to avoid contamination from spilling.

5. _____All specimens should be double bagged—in a plastic bag or wrap and then in a paper bag.

6. _____It is usually easier for the client to expel sputum for a specimen in the early morning after arising.

7. _____Completely fill the urine specimen container to have enough urine for examination.

8. _____Wear gloves when collecting specimens only when you think that you may spill the specimens.

9. _____Collect 5 oz of stool for a specimen.

10. _____When collecting a 24-hour urine specimen starting at 3 PM on Thursday, place both the first specimen voided at 3 PM on Thursday and the final specimen voided at 3 PM on Friday into the container.

CROSSWORD PUZZLE

Directions: Complete the crossword puzzle by identifying the important terms found in Chapter 16.

Across

2. Type of urine specimen

4. Semisolid waste from the large intestine

7. Specimens are sent here

9. Produced by the kidneys

10. Short, pointed blades

11. Organisms that live in or on another organism

Down

1. Determining the substances present in a specimen

3. Dirty; containing pathogens

5. Specimen is placed in this object

6. Stones formed in the body

8. Worn when handling specimens

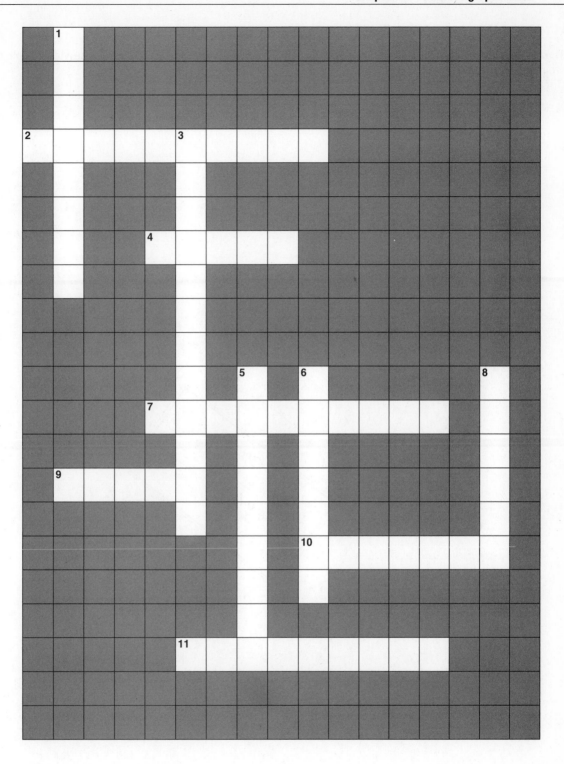

WHAT NEEDS TO BE CORRECTED?

Directions: In the figures that follow, problems with specimen collection are shown. In the space provided, explain what you would correct in each picture.

1. (Figure 16-1)

    A. What's wrong?

    _____

    B. Correction:

    _____

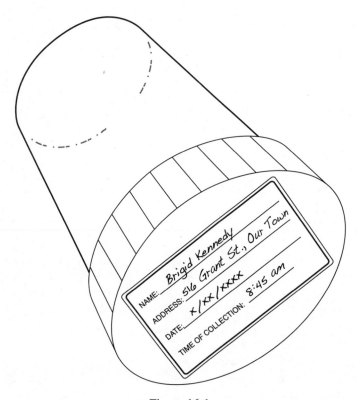

NAME: Brigid Kennedy
ADDRESS: 516 Grant St., Our Town
DATE: x/xx/xxxx
TIME OF COLLECTION: 8:45 am

Figure 16-1

2. (Figure 16-2)

   A. What's wrong?
   _____

   B. Correction:
   _____

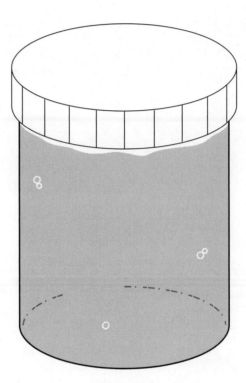

Figure 16-2

3. (Figure 16-3)

   A. What's wrong?
   _____

   B. Correction:
   _____

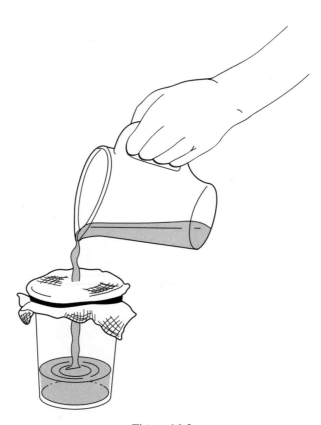

Figure 16-3

4. (Figure 16-4)

    A. What's wrong?

    _____

    B. Correction:

    _____

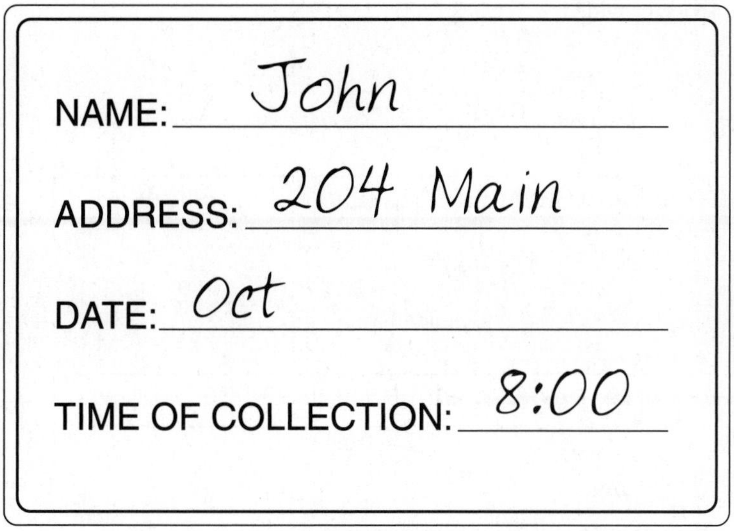

NAME: _John_____

ADDRESS: _204 Main_____

DATE: _Oct_____

TIME OF COLLECTION: _8:00___

Figure 16-4

17 Measuring Vital Signs

READING THE THERMOMETER

Directions: Below are several drawings of thermometers (Figure 17-1, *A* through *F*). Read each thermometer, and then write your reading in the space provided.

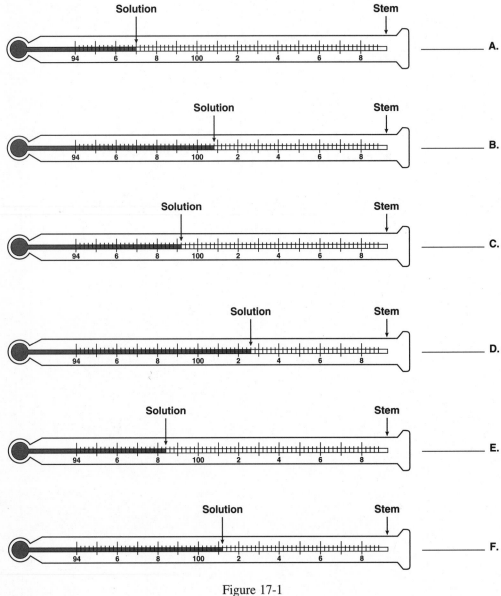

Figure 17-1

READING THE DIAL OF THE BLOOD PRESSURE CUFF

Directions: Below are several drawings of blood pressure cuff dials (Figure 17-2, *A* through *D*). Read each dial's indicator, and then write your reading in the space provided.

A. Blood pressure reading: _____

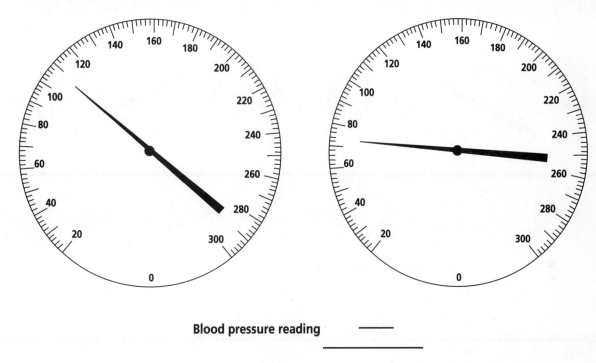

Blood pressure reading _____

Figure 17-2, *A*

B. Blood pressure reading: _____

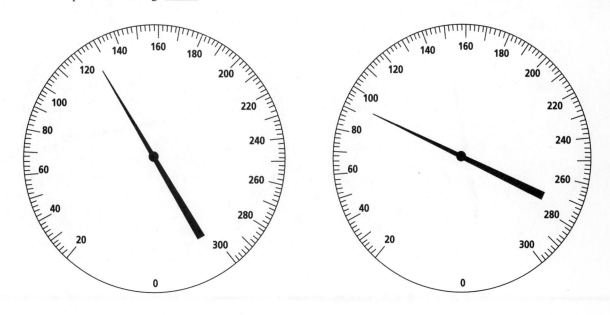

Blood pressure reading _____

Figure 17-2, *B*

C. Blood pressure reading: _____

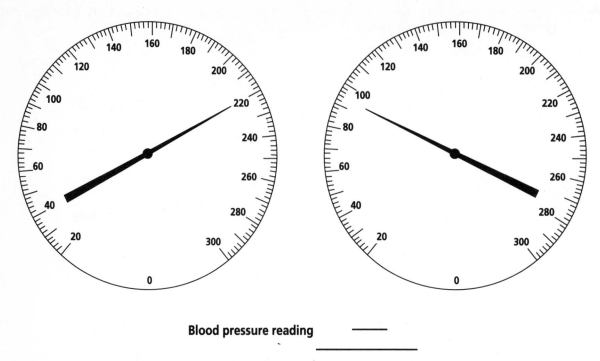

Blood pressure reading _____
_____

Figure 17-2, *C*

D. Blood pressure reading: _____

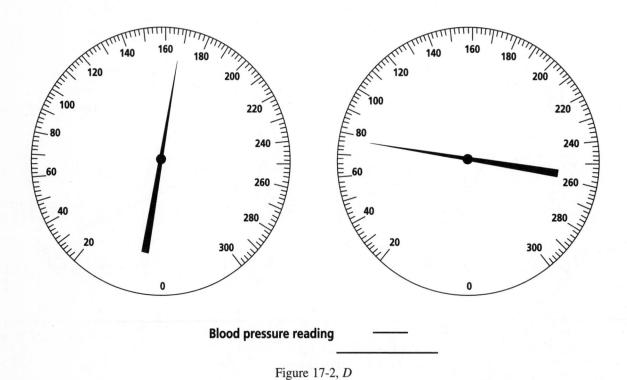

Blood pressure reading _____
_____

Figure 17-2, *D*

MATCHING

Directions: Match each term listed in Column A with its correct definition in Column B.

Column A

A. Chestpiece

B. Axillary

C. Inhalation

D. Radial artery

E. Systole

F. Stethoscope

G. Exhalation

H. Blood pressure

I. Diastole

J. Thermometer

K. Brachial artery

L. Dial

M. Hypertension

N. Vital signs

O. Pulse rate

Column B

1. _____Measures body heat

2. _____High blood pressure

3. _____Blood vessel used to measure blood pressure

4. _____Part of blood pressure cuff that shows numbers from 20 to 300 and has a pointer

5. _____Resting part of heart beat

6. _____Part of stethoscope

7. _____Temperature, pulse, respirations, and blood pressure

8. _____Contracting part of the heart beat

9. _____Removing carbon dioxide

10. _____Instrument used to hear beats in 1 minute

11. _____Number of heart beats in 1 minute

12. _____In the armpit

13. _____Located on palm side of the wrist at base of thumb

14. _____Measurement of force of blood against wall of an artery

15. _____Breathing in oxygen

REPORTING VITAL SIGNS

Directions: Listed below are several recordings of vital signs. Review this list, and, in the space provided, place an "X" beside the ones that you would report to your supervisor.

1. _____T: 103.2° F (O) (39.5° C)

2. _____P: 72, regular

3. _____T: 98.6° F (O) (37° C)

4. _____R: 10, with wheezing and pain

5. _____P: 123, weak

6. _____T: 99.5° F (T) (37.5° C)

7. _____BP: $\frac{118}{70}$

8. _____BP: $\frac{220}{94}$

9. _____BP: $\frac{70}{30}$

10. _____R: 16, periods of no breathing followed by rapid breathing

11. _____T: 99.6° F (O) (37.5° C)

12. _____P: 69, irregular

13. _____T: 96.8° F (A) (36° C)

14. _____T: 100.6° F (R) (38.1° C)

15. _____T: 102.2° F (O) (39° C)

COMPLETION

Directions: Fill in the blanks to complete each sentence.

1. Vital signs give important information about the body processes of _____, _____, and heat _____.

2. Take the client's vital signs when the client is _____.

3. Factors that cause vital signs to increase are _____, _____, and _____.

4. Heat leaves the body by means of _____ and _____.

5. It is 9:30 AM, and your client has just had a big cup of hot coffee. You should take the oral temperature at _____.

6. Have the client hold the thermometer in the mouth for _____ minutes before you remove and read the thermometer.

7. To read the thermometer, hold it at _____ level.

8. Remove the electronic thermometer and read the digital display window when you hear the _____.

9. Read the _____ dot to change color on the disposable thermometer.

10. Your client has diarrhea. Do not take a _____ temperature.

11. The normal systolic pressure in an adult is _____. The normal diastolic pressure in an adult is _____.

12. The normal range of TPRs in adults is:

    T (O): _____

    P: _____

    R: _____

13. Before and after using the stethoscope, clean the earpieces and the chestpiece to prevent the _____ of _____.

14. Shake down the oral thermometer to _____ before placing it under the client's tongue.

15. When cleaning the rectal thermometer, begin at the _____, and then wipe _____ toward the _____. Use a _____ motion.

16. Do not use your _____ to take your client's pulse.

17. You begin to take your client's pulse at 10:35 AM. You finish taking this pulse at _____ AM. You continue holding the pulse while you count respirations. You finish counting the respirations at _____ AM.

18 Special Procedures

SITUATIONS

Directions: Listed below are four situations you may experience as a home care aide. Read each situation, and then answer the questions in the space provided.

1. Olga has a chronic respiratory disease. She has difficulty breathing, and she receives oxygen by nasal cannula. While giving Olga a bed bath, you notice that the skin above her ears and around her nostrils is reddened where the plastic tubing comes in contact with these areas. Olga's lips are chapped, and she complains that her mouth is always dry.

   A. List at least three activities that you can perform to make Olga more comfortable.

   _____

   _____

   _____

   _____

   _____

   B. As a home care aide, you know that oxygen is one of the three ingredients that are needed for a fire. List five safety precautions to keep in mind when Olga is receiving oxygen.

   _____

   _____

   _____

   _____

   _____

2. You have been caring for Moishe, a 79-year-old man with diabetes, for several months. In addition to light house-keeping duties, his care plan includes the following:
   • Apply a clean, dry dressing to the reddened area of the lower left leg daily.
   • Apply warm soaks to the left foot for 20 minutes daily.

   A. List four signs that you will watch for when applying the warm soaks.

   _____

   _____

   _____

   _____

   _____

   B. How frequently will you check for these signs? Why?

   _____

   _____

   _____

   _____

   _____

C. When removing the tape on Moishe's dressing, you notice that his skin is very red. You also notice that there is a small amount of greenish drainage on the dressing. List two actions that you will take.

_____

_____

_____

3. Genevieve has severe arthritis. She lives with her daughter and her three grandchildren, who are all less than 5 years old. During your past two visits, Genevieve's daughter has complained about the time that it takes for her to care for her mother, including giving her mother a vitamin B_{12} injection: "If only her hands and eyesight were better, Mama could take care of herself and give herself the shot, too. These kids take a lot of my time." Today, as you finish giving Genevieve her shower, her daughter says, "Let me teach you how to give the vitamin shot. It's really very easy to do. You know how much Mama and I trust you. Besides, vitamins are not drugs, so you can give them. If I can do it, you certainly can do it even better."

A. What is your response to Genevieve's daughter?

_____

_____

_____

_____

_____

B. What will you do?

_____

4. Your client, Mrs. Choi, had problems with her heart and her circulation, especially in her legs. The care plan indicates that you are to assist Mrs. Choi with taking her heart medication and to help her to put on her elastic stockings after the bed bath. Mrs. Choi is usually not a complainer, but today she tells you about the severe cramps that she has been having in her legs during the night: "I didn't want to wake up my husband; he needs his sleep. Please don't tell anyone about this, I'm sure they'll go away."

A. What is your response to Mrs. Choi?

_____

_____

_____

_____

B. What will you do?

_____

C. When you remove the cap on Mrs. Choi's medication bottle, you notice that the pills are discolored and are crumbling. What two actions will you take?

_____

_____

_____

_____

PROCEDURES

Directions: Listed below are three special procedures that may be performed by the home care aide. For each procedure, review the steps that are listed, and then number them in the correct order.

1. Giving a sitz bath:

   ___Ask the client to void.

   ___Place the sitz bowl so that the drainage holes are at the back of the toilet.

   ___Ask the client to remove and discard any dressings or pads that are being worn. Assist with this process, if needed.

   ___Fill half of the plastic sitz bowl with warm water (94° to 98° F [34° to 37° C]).

   ___Dry the area, and then reapply the dressing or pad, if necessary.

   ___Instruct the client to open the clamp of the water bag to let warmer water into the bowl.

2. Applying hot compresses:

   ___Wring out the compress, and apply it to the area.

   ___Fill the basin or container ½ to ⅔ full of water at 105° to 115° F (40.5° to 46.1° C).

   ___Check the client's skin every 10 minutes for danger signs.

   ___Cover the compress quickly with plastic wrap.

   ___Place the waterproof protector pad under the body part to which the compress is to be applied.

   ___Put on gloves.

3. Applying an elastic stocking:

   ___Place the foot of the stocking over the client's toes, foot, and heel.

   ___Put the client in a supine position.

   ___Record what you have done.

   ___Adjust the stocking to fit smoothly, without folds or wrinkles.

   ___Turn the stocking inside out down to the heel.

   ___Fit the client's foot into the heel and toe portions of the stocking.

4. Assisting with transdermal disks:

   ___Have the client remove and discard the old disk into a waste container.

   ___Record what you have done.

   ___Observe as the client applies the new disk to the skin surface.

   ___Ask the client to a select site for the new disk.

   ___Wash the skin that had been covered by the old disk.

   ___Obtain materials.

MATCHING

Directions: Match each term listed in Column B with its correct definition in Column A.

Column A

_____1. Medications that can be bought without a prescription

_____2. Gas needed by all cells in the body

_____3. Small gelatin container that holds medication

_____4. Inside a vein

_____5. Absorbed through the skin

_____6. A two-pronged device that delivers oxygen; short prongs are inserted into the client's nostrils

_____7. Solid forms of medication for insertion into a body cavity

_____8. A blood clot

_____9. Small cylinders containing a drug that is inhaled in specifically measured (metered) doses

_____10. A blood clot that travels through the circulatory system until it lodges in a distant blood vessel

Column B

A. Capsule

B. Transdermal

C. Suppositories

D. Metered-dose inhaler (MDI)

E. Intravenous

F. OTC

G. Oxygen

H. Nasal cannula

I. Thrombus

J. Embolus

TRUE OR FALSE

Directions: In the space provided, mark the statement "T" for true or "F" for false. If the statement is false, change it to make it true.

1. ___Medications are substances that are used for the treatment of a disease or illness.

2. ___Over-the-counter drugs can be purchased without a prescription.

3. ___Oral medications should be taken with a small sip of water.

4. ___Clients place sublingual tablets under the tongue.

5. ___Topical medications and transdermal disks are both applied to the skin.

6. ___The method by which medication is taken is called the *route*.

7. ___The amount of medication to be taken is called the *dose*.

8. ___When one dose is forgotten or omitted, it's OK for the client to take a double dose the next time.

9. ___If your client says that the tablets are the wrong shape and color, tell him or her to take them anyway.

10. ___If your client does not take a medication, notify your supervisor.

11. ___Record if a medication is not taken (or omitted) and why.

12. ___Unused medications should be saved, because they might be needed again.

13. ___Vaseline may be used to lubricate a rectal suppository.

14. ___Transdermal disks are usually applied to the chest or the upper arm.

15. ___Older adults are at great risk for burns from applications of heat.

16. ___When applying heat or cold, be sure to check the client's skin every 30 minutes.

17. ___Hot compresses are an example of moist heat.

18. ___Sitz baths may be given by having the client soak in the bathtub.

19. ___Oxygen is a drug, and it is part of the client's treatment or therapy.

20. ___"No Smoking" and "Oxygen in Use" signs are placed on the front door of a residence where oxygen is being used.

21. ___Home care aides may regulate the flow of intravenous fluids.

22. ___A blood clot is called a *thrombus*.

23. ___Elastic stockings should be removed three times a day to check the color and warmth of the client's legs and feet.

24. ___The improper application of elastic stockings or elastic bandages can block circulation and cause damage to tissues.

25. ___Elastic bandages should be applied as tightly as possible.

WHAT NEEDS TO BE CORRECTED?

Directions: In the figures that follow, problems with personal care are shown. In the space provided, explain what you would correct in each picture.

1. (Figure 18-1)

   A. What's wrong?

   _____

   B. Correction:

   _____

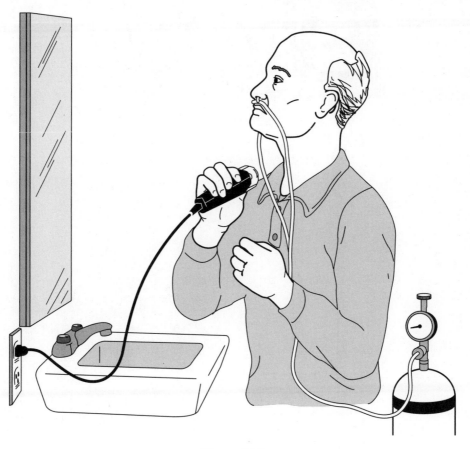

Figure 18-1

2. (Figure 18-2)

   A. What's wrong?

   _____

   B. Correction:

   _____

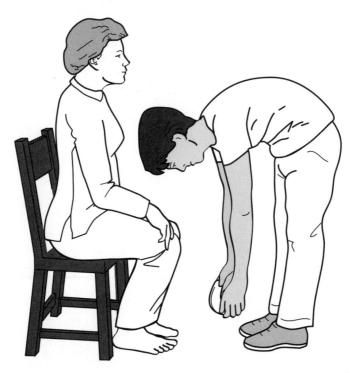

Figure 18-2

3. (Figure 18-3)

A. What's wrong?

_____

B. Correction:

_____

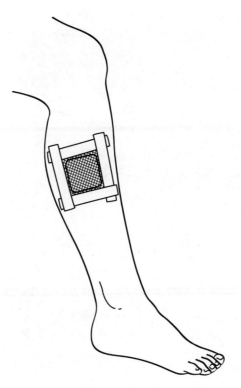

Figure 18-3

4. (Figure 18-4)

A. What's wrong?

_____

B. Correction:

_____

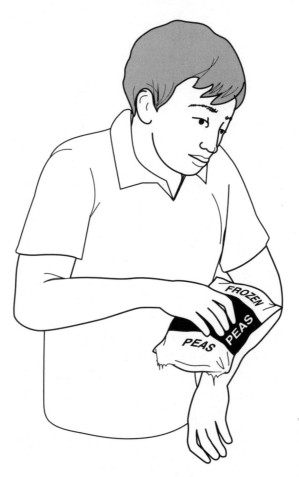

Figure 18-4

19 Caring for Older Adults

TRUE OR FALSE

Directions: In the space provided, mark the statement "T" for true or "F" for false. If the statement is false, change it to make it true.

1. ___Aging begins when a person is 65 years old.

2. ___Incontinence is normal for clients who are more than 80 years old.

3. ___There are more older women than older men.

4. ___As normal aging progresses, the older person's personality will surely change.

5. ___Mental confusion is a normal part of growing old.

6. ___Try to change the subject when your client begins to talk about the "old times."

7. ___The need for home care will decrease in the future, because the life span of older adults is decreasing.

8. ___There are three categories of older adults: the young old, the middle old, and the oldest old.

9. ___The rate at which we age depends on one factor only: our heredity.

10. ___Loneliness is a common experience for many older adults.

11. ___Older adults can't learn new things.

12. ___Accepting oneself as an aging person is one of the adjustments that older adults need to make.

13. ___The portion of the population that is growing at the most rapid rate is made of individuals who are 65 to 75 years old.

14. ___You do not need to explain what you are going to do for the older adult; he or she won't understand what you are saying.

15. ___Twenty percent of older adults are cared for in institutions.

NORMAL CONDITIONS OF AGING

Directions: Describe a way that you can help your client to cope with each of the normal conditions of aging that are listed.

1. Difficulty adjusting to a dark room

_____

_____

2. Forgetting where eyeglasses were placed

_____

_____

3. Dry skin

_____

_____

4. Dry mouth

_____

_____

5. Feeling cold

_____

_____

6. Occasional constipation

_____

_____

7. Shortness of breath with increased activity

_____

_____

8. Feeling anxious about changes in routine

_____

_____

9. Having an urgent need to void

_____

_____

10. Feeling bloated

_____

_____

11. Rapid heart beat when under stress

_____

_____

12. Trouble adjusting to depths (going up and down stairs)

_____

_____

13. Having trouble understanding what you are saying

_____

_____

14. Thick, hard toenails

_____

_____

15. Experiencing unsteadiness when rising suddenly from a chair

_____

_____

SITUATIONS

Directions: Answer the questions about the following situations:

1. Mrs. Edwards, who is 75 years old, has recently returned from the rehabilitation center, where she learned to walk after fracturing her hip. Today, her daughter, who is visiting for the day, greets you at the door and asks you to come into the kitchen. You can smell the odor of stale beer in the apartment. The daughter closes the door and whispers, "I'm really worried about Mom. She's always liked a few beers while watching television at night, but now she's drinking a six pack a day or more. Lately, she refuses to eat any meals; she just sits and drinks that beer and eats pretzels. Mom says that it's none of my business. Will you tell her not to drink? She won't listen to me." Later, while cleaning Mrs. Edwards' room, you notice that there are three cases of beer under her bed.

A. How will you answer the daughter's question?

B. What will you do with the three cases of beer?

C. What will you do?

2. Magdalena is a frail 80-year-old woman who speaks very little English. She lives with her nephew and his wife, and this is your first visit to their home. Magdalena's care plan indicates that you are to help her to take a shower, dress, and walk and that you need to change her bed linens. Magdalena's nephew greets you at the door and appears to be very upset. He says, "Last week, Auntie peed on the new sofa in the living room. Now, it's all ruined. She's never done anything like this before. We know that she did it on purpose, just to get even with us for not taking her to visit her grandson." He continues, "My wife is so angry that she locks Auntie in her bedroom so that she won't ruin the rest of the furniture!" As the nephew unlocks Magdalena's bedroom door, you can hear Magdalena crying in bed. She speaks to you in Spanish. You do not understand what she is saying, but you know that she is terribly upset. The bed linens are dirty with urine and feces, and it appears that they have not been changed for several days.

A. How will you respond to Magdalena?

B. What will you do?

_____

_____

_____

_____

_____

C. What will you record?

_____

_____

_____

_____

_____

D. What will you say to Magdalena's nephew?

_____

_____

_____

_____

_____

3. Mr. Lewis is 79 years old, and he has lived alone since his wife died 3 years ago. Recently, he was hospitalized for a heart condition. You have been caring for him three times a week for the past 2 weeks. Today, you notice that he is confused and that he is wearing dirty pajamas. In the kitchen, there is a stack of dirty dishes in the sink, and there is an uneaten meal on the table that was left by a Meals On Wheels volunteer the previous day.

List four activities that you would perform to help Mr. Lewis.

A. _____

B. _____

C. _____

D. _____

20 Caring for Mothers, Infants, and Children

MATCHING

Directions: Match each term listed in Column B with its correct definition in Column A.

Column A

____1. Space covered by tough membranes between bones of infant's skull

____2. Discharge from the vagina after birth

____3. Colored, circular area surrounding the nipple

____4. Educated guess about the probable outcome of an illness

____5. First 6 weeks following the birth of a baby

____6. System of rules that governs the way we act

____7. Emotional attachment between infant and parents, especially the mother

____8. The completion of 37-40 weeks of pregnancy

____9. Normal reaction infants have that makes them begin to suck when their cheeks are stroked

___10. Enlarged veins in the rectum or anus

Column B

A. Bond

B. Hemorrhoids

C. Fontanel

D. Discipline

E. Lochia

F. Full term

G. Prognosis

H. Rooting reflex

I. Areola

J. Postpartum period

RECOGNIZING NORMAL AND ABNORMAL CONDITIONS IN THE MOTHER

Directions: Review the following list of observations. Place an "X" beside those conditions that you would immediately report to your supervisor.

1. ____Mother complains of discomfort in the perineal area

2. ____Weight loss of 19 lbs (8.6 kg) on the 10th day after delivery

3. ____Three pads are used within 1 hour and contain a large number of blood clots

4. ____Hemorrhoids in the anal area

5. ____Cracked skin around the left nipple

6. ____Elevated temperature (101° F [38.4° C], oral)

7. ____Mother complains of tenderness in the calf muscle of the right leg

8. ____Brownish lochia on the ninth day after delivery

9. ____Mother says, "I feel so sad today, I just want to cry."

10. ____Breasts are painful and hot to the touch

11. ____Mother refuses to drink fluids because "My breasts will dry up faster."

12. ____Vaginal discharge has a foul odor

13. ____Lochia is scant and cream-colored on the 20th day after delivery

14. ____Mother eats only skim milk, gelatin, and dry crackers because she says, "I want to lose all the weight I gained. I hate being fat!"

15. ____Tender breasts on the third day after delivery

16. ____No bowel movements for 5 days

17. ____Mother not interested in surroundings, withdrawn, and refusing to eat

18. ____Swelling and redness around the abdominal incision (after cesarean birth)

19. ____Mother complains of being exhausted on the second and third days after delivery

20. ____Mother worries about being able to care for the infant properly

SITUATIONS

Directions: Answer the questions about the following situations:

1. You are scheduled to visit Amanda, a 17-year-old single mother. Her baby, Jeffrey, is now 8 days old. Both mother and baby are well and healthy. The professional nurse has been visiting Amanda to help her learn how to care for Jeffrey. Today, you find Amanda lying on her bed and sobbing. Between sobs, she tells you, "I'll never learn to be a good mother. The baby cries all the time, and I can't get him to breast-feed right away. I never thought being a mother would be such hard work! Where is my boyfriend to help me?"

   A. How will you communicate with Amanda?

   _____

   _____

   _____

   _____

   _____

   B. What will you do?

   _____

   _____

   _____

   _____

   _____

2. Just after Yolanda Potts brought her new baby home from the hospital, her older child, Johnny, says, "I don't like that baby. She stinks!" Johnny is 4 years old. He has been toilet trained for a year, but he now becomes incontinent. Yolanda tells the home care aide, "I am so tired with a new baby. Johnny is acting like a baby, too. I could just smack him."

   List three things that you would do.
   A. _____

   _____

   B. _____

   _____

   C. _____

   _____

TRUE OR FALSE

Directions: In the space provided, mark the statement "T" for true or "F" for false. If the statement is false, change it to make it true.

1. ____An infant is given a tub bath after the umbilical stump falls off.

2. ____Newborn infants are awake for most of the day.

3. ____Sleeping infants should be placed on their backs.

4. ____The stool of a breast-fed infant is dark brown and formed.

5. ____Infants are burped only at the end of every feeding.

6. ____The first breast "milk" is known as *colostrum.*

7. ____Infants chill quickly, and their hands and feet become bluish and cold.

8. ____The umbilical stump falls off after 2 weeks.

9. ____Newborn infants eat four times a day.

10. ____Bottles of formula may be warmed in the microwave.

11. ____Test the temperature of baby bath water on your elbow.

12. ____Mothers should be in a comfortable position when they are breast-feeding or bottle-feeding.

13. ____Children do not react to stress.

14. ____Follow (client's) family rules regarding discipline.

15. ____Children often use nonverbal communication as a means of expressing an emotional response to stress.

OBSERVATION

Directions: Review the following list of observations of a normal newborn infant. Place an "X" beside those conditions that you would immediately report to your supervisor.

1. ____Yellow skin

2. ____Bluish and cold hands and feet

3. ____Spitting up small amounts of feedings when burped

4. ____Crying and fussing every 3 hours

5. ____Wet diaper at every feeding

6. ____Sleeping most of the time

7. ____Crying constantly; cannot be comforted

8. ____Limp; hardly moves or cries

9. ____Has several yellow bowel movements each day

10. ____Cries during bath

21 Caring for Clients With Mental Illness

CROSSWORD PUZZLE

Directions: Complete the crossword puzzle by identifying the important terms found in Chapter 21.

Across

2. Use of violent or abusive behavior to cope with anxiety

3. A sudden, uncontrollable urge

4. Feeling of being extremely frightened and unable to move

8. Fearful about real or imagined threats to a person's well-being

9. Returning to behaviors, thoughts, or feelings used at an earlier stage of development

10. False beliefs held as true, despite evidence to the contrary

Down

1. Term used to describe the misuse of chemical substances that leads to an emotional or physical dependence

5. Mental state in which a client is disoriented about time, place, or person

6. A disorder characterized by feelings of extreme sadness and hopelessness

7. Sensory perception (things seen, heard, felt, and smelled) that aren't actually there

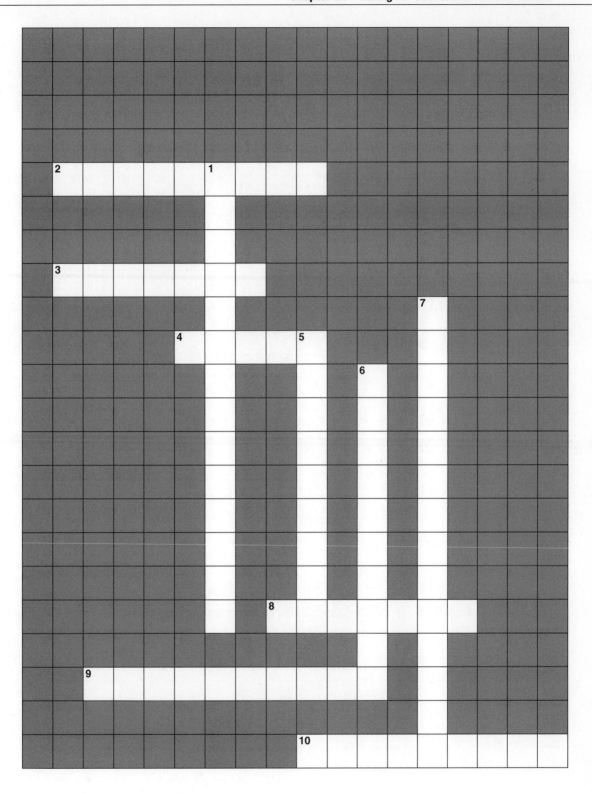

SITUATIONS

Directions: Fill in the blanks about the following situations:

1. Your client is overactive and constantly pacing back and forth throughout the home. How will you meet the following needs?

    A. Food and fluid needs:

    _____

    _____

    _____

    B. Elimination needs:

    _____

    _____

    _____

    C. Hygiene and grooming needs:

    _____

    _____

    _____

    _____

    _____

2. George's wife tells you that he has been very confused. He tries to put on his socks after putting on his shoes; he begins to get ready for bed at 9 AM, thinking that it is evening; and he tries to drink the dishwashing detergent, thinking that it is soda. How can you help George with each of these problems?

    _____

    _____

    _____

    _____

    _____

3. How will you meet your client's needs that result from the following behaviors:

    A. Refuses to eat or drink fluids prepared for him because he thinks that they are "poison":

    _____

    _____

    _____

    _____

    B. Carries on conversations with people when there are no people present:

    _____

    _____

    _____

    _____

C. Refuses to take his medications because "they are poison, too":

_____

_____

_____

_____

4. Your client is depressed and sad most of the day. He cries easily, and he tells you, "I'm too tired to even lift a fork or glass to feed myself." He also tells you that he doesn't even have the energy to go to the bathroom.

How will you meet the following needs?

A. Food and fluid needs:

_____

_____

_____

B. Elimination needs:

_____

_____

_____

He says, "I can't stand feeling like this anymore; maybe I should just end it all."

C. What should you say?

_____

_____

_____

D. What should you do?

_____

_____

_____

5. Your elderly client is very confused. She sometimes gets out of the house, stands on the front porch, and takes off all of her clothes. Other times, she removes her clothing and stands by the window exposing herself.

A. What measures may prevent this type of behavior?

_____

_____

_____

_____

_____

B. What can you do if this does happen?

_____

_____

_____

_____

_____

6. Your client is recovering from injuries that he received during an automobile accident. He uses a wheelchair to get around his apartment, and he needs assistance with his activities of daily living, especially hygiene and grooming. When you reach into the top drawer of his bureau to get his electric razor, you discover a syringe and several small cellophane bags that contain a white powder.

   A. What should you do?

   _____

   _____

   _____

   _____

7. Your client's daughter says, "I can't stand my mother since she got sick and I have to take care of her. The only thing that helps is this." She lights a marijuana cigarette. She invites you to join her, saying, "Have some, dearie, it'll make life a lot easier."

   A. What should you say?

   _____

   _____

   _____

   _____

   B. What should you do?

   _____

   _____

   _____

   _____

22 Caring for Clients With Illnesses Requiring Home Care

CLIENT CONDITIONS

Directions: You are caring for eight clients during the week. Each client has one of the following conditions. Below each condition, describe two activities that you will perform to assist your client.

1. Wandering

_____

_____

_____

2. Fatigue

_____

_____

_____

3. Difficulty swallowing

_____

_____

_____

4. Pain

_____

_____

_____

5. Paralysis or weakness on the right side of the body

_____

_____

_____

6. Diarrhea

_____

_____

_____

7. Difficulty breathing

_____

_____

_____

8. Sores in the mouth

_____

_____

_____

SITUATIONS

Directions: Fill in the blanks about the following situation:

1. Mrs. Gable's daughter, Susan, had been worried about her mother for more than a year. Susan noticed that her mother became more forgetful and confused and that her mother's personality seemed to change, too. These were real concerns, especially because Mrs. Gable lived alone. One evening, as Susan entered the front door of Mrs. Gable's home, she smelled something burning. In the kitchen, her mother had placed a frozen dinner—carton and all—into a frying pan and turned on the stove. Susan arrived just in time to put out the fire. The next week, Susan took her mother to the doctor for a checkup. After further testing, Mrs. Gable was diagnosed as having Alzheimer's disease. Now, Mrs. Gable lives with Susan, and you live next door to both of them.

A. Susan asks your advice about making her home safer for her mother. List five suggestions that you will give her.
   1. _____
   2. _____
   3. _____
   4. _____
   5. _____

B. Mrs. Gable hides her eyeglasses, and then she can't find them. How will you advise Susan to handle this situation?

_____

_____

_____

_____

C. Mrs. Gable cannot remember the names of her daughter, her son-in-law, and her two grandchildren. This makes her very upset. What will you suggest to help remember their names?

_____

_____

_____

_____

D. Mrs. Gable forgets to go to the bathroom and soils her underpants frequently. Sometimes she becomes confused and doesn't know where the bathroom is located, and then she cries. What advice can you give?

_____
_____
_____
_____
_____

E. Susan says that she heard about an Alzheimer's support group that meets each week in a nearby church hall. She asks you about the benefits of joining such a group. How will you reply?

_____
_____
_____
_____
_____

2. Mr. Yancy has been receiving a series of radiation treatments at the local medical center after undergoing cancer surgery. He returns home after each treatment. The day after his treatment, he is exhausted and has no appetite. A transdermal patch placed on his upper arm provides him with medication to help relieve the severe pain in his back. During each visit, you help Mr. Yancy to take a partial bath at the bathroom sink, and you prepare his lunch and perform various housekeeping duties.

A. How will you help Mr. Yancy with the partial bath?

_____
_____
_____
_____
_____

B. There are markings on Mr. Yancy's lower back where the radiation treatments are given. How will you care for this area?

_____
_____
_____
_____
_____

C. What will you do to encourage Mr. Yancy to eat?

_____
_____
_____
_____
_____

D. List four conditions that you will report to your supervisor.

_____

_____

_____

_____

_____

3. Your client, Fernando, has acquired immunodeficiency syndrome. He lives alone in a two-room apartment, and he looks forward to your visit each day. Fernando spends a lot of time in bed because he has very little energy. In addition, he has the following symptoms:
   - Cough; brings up blood-tinged sputum
   - No appetite
   - Diarrhea about twice a week
   - 20-lb weight loss over the past 6 weeks
   - Bleeding gums
   - Swelling of the legs and ankles

Fernando's care plan includes giving him a complete bed bath, encouraging his fluid intake, and keeping his feet elevated when he is out of bed.

A. Describe five special precautions that you will take to control infection when caring for Fernando. Explain your reasons.

_____

_____

_____

_____

_____

B. You notice that there are reddened areas on Fernando's elbows, heels, and lower back. What will you do?

_____

_____

_____

_____

C. When preparing meals for Fernando, list three precautions that you will take to prevent infection.

_____

_____

_____

_____

_____

D. One day, while you are caring for Fernando, his sister comes to visit. She says to you, "You're very brave to be caring for my brother. Don't you worry that you'll get AIDS from him?" How will you answer this question?

_____

_____

_____

_____

_____

E. Fernando's sister also tells you that she and her brother were always very fond of each other. "We were always hugging. Now, it's different. He's so sick; I'm afraid to even touch him." What is your response?

_____

_____

_____

_____

_____

4. Your client, Sara Turner, had her gallbladder removed. She has returned home after one night in the hospital. She has a tube in her abdomen that is draining green liquid into a collecting bag, which is almost full. She needs to cough, but she is afraid to do so. She complains about pain in the area of the drain. What would you do about the following?

A. The drainage bag is almost full:

_____

_____

B. Her fear of coughing:

_____

_____

C. Pain in the area of the drainage tube:

_____

_____

5. After a cerebrovascular accident, Mrs. Potts was transferred to a rehabilitation center, where she learned to walk using a walker. She still has some difficulty chewing and swallowing, and she doesn't always remember the correct names of things. She is easily frustrated, and she cries when she is unable to do certain things. How can you help Mrs. Potts with the following?

A. Safe ambulation:

_____

_____

_____

_____

_____

B. Adequate nutrition:

_____

_____

_____

_____

_____

C. Communication:

_____

_____

_____

_____

D. Emotional support:

_____

_____

_____

_____

6. Mr. Fugil was admitted to the medical center in an unconscious state. Tests revealed a very high blood glucose level, and diabetes mellitus was diagnosed. When Mr. Fugil was discharged, you were assigned to assist him, because he was very weak and needed help with personal care for a short time. You discover that Mr. Fugil is not following the prescribed diet. He snacks on cake, cookies, cheese, and crackers, and he has ice cream for dessert every night. He refuses to test his blood glucose, and he also refuses to take his insulin; he says he doesn't like to "stick" himself. What should you do?

_____

_____

_____

_____

TRUE OR FALSE

Directions: In the space provided, mark the statement "T" for true or "F" for false. If the statement is false, change it to make it true.

1. ____Another name for stroke is *cerebrovascular accident.*

2. ____Clients with chronic obstructive pulmonary disease have difficulty breathing.

3. ____Edema is the swelling of the tissues, and it is common with cardiovascular disease.

4. ____Cancer is the second leading cause of death in the United States.

5. ____Cancer treatment causes no side effects or problems.

6. ____Parkinson's disease is an acute illness that affects young adults.

7. ____Clients with multiple sclerosis often experience fatigue.

8. ____Postoperative clients are at risk for infection.

9. ____Reasoning with an Alzheimer's client will help him or her to understand what is happening.

10. ____An identification bracelet is important for the Alzheimer's client who wanders.

11. ____Clients with circulatory problems tire easily.

12. ____Human immunodeficiency virus causes AIDS.

13. ____Diarrhea, malnutrition, and wasting are serious problems for clients with AIDS.

14. ____Standard (universal) precautions are used only when caring for clients with AIDS.

15. ____Clients with AIDS should not handle soiled cat litter or other animal bedding.

16. ____The term *arthritis* means "inflammation of the joints."

17. ____A client with a cast can take a tub bath.

18. ____It is normal for a client with a casted arm to have cold, blue fingers that he or she cannot move.

19. ____Always wear gloves when handling any client's body fluids.

20. ____Encourage clients to do as much as possible for themselves according to their condition.

21. ____The home care aide may change sterile surgical dressings.

22. ____"Phantom limb pain" after an amputation is all in the client's imagination.

23. ____Clients with low energy levels should not be rushed through their activities of daily living.

24. ____Clients with poor appetites should be given big meals that include lots of food.

25. ____Many clients with chronic illnesses have low self-images; they are often frustrated and discouraged.

23 Caring for the Client at the End of Life

COMPLETION

Directions: Fill in the blanks to complete each sentence.

1. Clients' emotional responses to dying include _____, _____, _____, _____, and _____.

2. A final illness from which a client is not expected to recover is called a _____ *illness* or an _____ *disease*.

3. A living will and durable power of attorney are examples of _____.

4. A program that cares for the dying client and his or her caregivers is called _____.

5. Two signs of approaching death are _____ and _____.

6. The last sense to leave the body is _____.

7. Care that is provided after death is called _____ *care*.

SITUATIONS

Directions: Fill in the blanks about the following situations:

1. Mr. Toomey has terminal cancer. He is no longer being treated for the disease, and he is being cared for in a hospice program. He asks you, "Am I going to die?" How would you respond?

_____

_____

_____

_____

_____

2. Your client is very sad and quiet. She sleeps most of the day, and she does not want any company. Her family is very upset; they feel that she has given up and that she does not want to get well. What would you do?

_____

_____

_____

_____

_____

3. Your client and his caregivers keep hoping for a miracle cure for the client's cancer. They read medical journals and search computer Web sites in the hope of learning about a cure. What is your feeling about their hope?

_____

_____

_____

_____

_____

4. Josephine tells you that you are stupid and that you do everything wrong. She says, "You don't even know how to comb my hair right." You have been caring for this hospice client for 4 weeks. How would you answer her?

_____
_____
_____
_____

5. Even though you knew that your client was going to die, when it happened, you were shocked. The next day, you feel very sad, and you cry about his death. How can you cope with these feelings?

_____
_____
_____
_____

6. Your client's wife tells you that, after her husband dies, the elders of her religious community will bathe and dress the body in preparation for immediate burial. What should you do?

_____
_____
_____
_____

7. The Weinberg family wants to say goodbye to their dying mother, but they say it's too late because she is already unconscious. What would you tell them?

_____
_____
_____
_____

24 Emergencies

COMPLETION

Directions: Fill in the blanks to complete each sentence.

1. The emergency telephone number to call in my area is _____.

2. Four questions that the dispatcher may ask when you report an emergency are _____, _____, _____, and _____.

3. The Four Cs of Emergency Care are _____, _____, _____, and _____.

4. First aid situations that increase the home care aide's risk for infection are _____, _____, and _____.

5. The four signs of a medical emergency that require immediate action are _____, _____, _____, and _____.

SITUATIONS (A)

Directions: For each of the emergency situations listed below, list four actions that you will perform in addition to calling for help.

1. The victim has severe bleeding from a wound on the right arm.
   A. _____
   B. _____
   C. _____
   D. _____

2. Victim appears gray and has cold, clammy skin; a weak, rapid pulse; and shallow respirations.
   A. _____
   B. _____
   C. _____
   D. _____

3. The client scalds his left hand while pouring boiling water from a pan on the stove. The area is very red, and there are blisters forming on the skin.
   A. _____
   B. _____
   C. _____
   D. _____

4. The client tells you that she feels like she is going to have a seizure.
   A. _____
   B. _____
   C. _____
   D. _____

5. The victim is not breathing, cannot speak, has his hands around his neck, and is sitting in a chair.
   A. _____
   _____
   B. _____
   _____
   C. _____
   _____
   D. _____
   _____

6. The client has fallen down the last three steps of the stairway. She is on her left side, and she complains of severe pain in her left leg and hip. Also, she cannot move her left wrist.
   A. _____
   B. _____
   C. _____
   D. _____

7. You are shopping at the local mall with your friend. Suddenly, he clutches his chest and says, "The pain is back. Now it's in my left arm, too."
   A. _____
   B. _____
   C. _____
   D. _____

SITUATIONS (B)

Directions: Read the following situations. In the space provided, answer the questions asked about each situation.
1. While walking from the bus stop to your client's apartment, a woman runs toward you. Her coat is on fire. What will you do first?

_____
_____
_____

2. Your aunt asks you to advise her about what items to buy for her family's first aid kit. List six items that you will recommend.

A. _____

B. _____

C. _____

D. _____

E. _____

F. _____

3. You find Louisa, a 3-year-old girl, in the bathroom drinking toilet bowl cleaner. List two actions that you will take.

A. _____

_____

B. _____

_____

Who will you call? What will you report?

_____

_____

_____

_____

4. Your client has been taken to the hospital by emergency medical services personnel after a medical emergency. What four pieces of information will you include when reporting the emergency to your agency and recording it?

A. _____

B. _____

C. _____

D. _____

25 Getting a Job and Keeping It

WANT AD

Directions: Read the want ad below, and then answer the questions about it.

CERTIFIED HOME CARE AIDES

ABC Home Care Agency, Inc., is currently expanding services.

Exp. pref'd. Cert. req. Car req.

*M-F + wknd

*Live-in work

*Excel pay + benefits

*Travel reim.

Email resume to ABCHC@noaddress.com

---

1. What do the following abbreviations mean?

   A. Exp. _____

   B. Pref'd. _____

   C. Cert. _____

   D. Req. _____

   E. Excel _____

   F. Reim. _____

2. What do the following terms mean?
   A. Travel reim.

   _____

   B. M-F + wknd

   _____

C. Live-in work

_____

_____

_____

D. Benefits

_____

_____

_____

3. Before e-mailing the ABC Home Care Agency about the want ad, how would you prepare?

A. _____

B. _____

THE JOB INTERVIEW

Directions: Answer the questions in the space provided.

1. Your appointment to be interviewed by the personnel manager of the ABC Home Care Agency is tomorrow at 1:30 PM. You should arrive at the agency no later than _____.
2. Complete the sample application form (Figure 25-1 on pp. 111–112).

APPLICATION FOR EMPLOYMENT
(Please print clearly)

Personal Information   **Date:** _____

Name _____
                    Last   First   Middle

Address _____
                    Street   City   State   Zip Code

Telephone _____ Social Security No. _____
            Area Code   Number

If under 18 years of age, do you have work permit?   ❏ Yes ❏ No

If not a U.S. citizen, do you have the right to remain permanently and work in the U.S.A.?   ❏ Yes ❏   No

    Alien Reg. No. _____

Employment Desired

Position applied for: _____

Shift you can work: ❏ Day   ❏ Evening   ❏ Either   Hours desired: ❏ Full time   ❏ Part time   ❏ Temporary

How did you learn of this opening? _____

Date you can start: _____
                            Month   Day   Year

Have you ever applied to this company before?   ❏ Yes ❏ No When _____

Have you ever worked for this company before?   ❏ Yes ❏ No
When _____ Supervisor _____

Reason for Leaving _____
_____

Education

	1 2 3 4 5 6 7 8	9 10 11 12	1 2 3 4
Highest grade completed (circle):	Grade School	High School	College

Name and location of last school attended _____

Vocational or trade training _____

Extracurricular
activities while in school _____

Area of specialization
or major interest _____

Professional organization memberships, honors received, volunteer or community service or other qualifications you have which
you feel are related to the position for which you are applying:

_____

_____

_____

_____

Form 3290R BRIGGS, Des Moines, IA 50306 (800) 247-2343 PRINTED IN U.S.A.   Rev. 4/92

Figure 25-1 (Courtesy Briggs Corporation, Des Moines, Iowa)

References

List three persons who know you well. Do not include relatives or former employers.

Name	Address	Phone	Years Acquainted With You

Former Employers

List below your work experience, starting with your present or last place of employment.

Date Employed	Name and Address of Employer	Name of Supervisor	Position(s) Held
from _____	_____	_____	start _____
to _____	_____	_____	finish _____
from _____	_____	_____	start _____
to _____	_____	_____	finish _____
from _____	_____	_____	start _____
to _____	_____	_____	finish _____
from _____	_____	_____	start _____
to _____	_____	_____	finish _____
from _____	_____	_____	start _____
to _____	_____	_____	finish _____

May we contact your present employer at this time?   ❑ Yes   ❑ No

Employment Understanding (Please Read and Sign)

This institution does not discriminate in hiring or any other decision on the basis of race, color, sex, citizenship, national origin, ancestry, Vietnam era veteran status, or on the basis of age or physical or mental disability unrelated to the ability to perform the work required. No question on this application is intended to secure information to be used for such discrimination.

I voluntarily give this institution the right to make a thorough investigation of my past employment and activities, agree to cooperate in such investigation and release from all liability or responsibility all persons, companies or corporations supplying such information. I consent to take the physical examination, and such future physical examinations as may be required by this institution at such times and places as the institution shall designate. I understand that an offer of employment may be contingent on passing the physical examination which relates to the essential duties I would be required to perform.

I understand that my employment is at will, and that either party is free to terminate the employment relationship at any time without cause. I also understand that my employment may be terminated for any misstatement or omission of fact appearing on this application form.

If employed, I will be required to complete an Employment Verification Form (1-9), and within three days show satisfactory evidence of identity and eligibility for employment.

_____   _____
Applicant's Signature   Date

Figure 25-1, cont'd

3. During the interview, the personnel manager, Ms. Hanson, explains the responsibilities of certified home care aides as employees of the ABC Home Care Agency. She discusses work hours, pay, and benefits. However, she has not discussed travel requirements or uniforms. What will you do?

_____

_____

_____

4. Ms. Hanson explains to you the rights of the ABC Home Care Agency. Under each right listed below, give two examples of how you will act to respect that right.

A. Right to expect that you will perform your duties properly:

1._____

2._____

B. Right to expect you to keep accurate records:

1._____

2._____

C. Right to expect you to use correct safety practices to protect yourself and your client:

1._____

2._____

D. Right to supervise and evaluate your performance:

1._____

2._____

5. Ms. Hanson also gives you information about your rights as an employee. Under each right listed below, give two examples of what your employer should do to respect that right.

A. Right to a safe working environment:

1._____

2._____

B. Right to be paid for the work that you perform:

1._____

2._____

C. Right to be supervised properly:

1._____

2._____

_____

D. Right to be evaluated regularly:

1._____

2._____

_____

6. Next to each behavior listed below, write "Yes" or "No" to indicate whether it is a correct action to take.

____A. Smoking

____B. Asking questions if you do not understand what the interviewer is saying

____C. Taking off your shoes because they are new and too tight

____D. Bringing your children with you

____E. Using your pen and paper to write down information that you want to remember

____F. Chewing gum

____G. Arriving early

____H. Thanking the interviewer for his or her time

____I. Keeping your cell phone handy in case you get a call during the interview

CROSSWORD PUZZLE

Directions: Complete the crossword puzzle by identifying the important terms found in Chapter 25.

Across

1. A person who helps students find employment

4. Health insurance, life insurance, and a prescription plan

6. To receive a copy of the personnel policies and to keep records of your attendance

8. Recognition by a government agency that an individual has met certain requirements

10. A formal meeting between an employer and a job applicant

11. Matches job seekers and potential employers

12. Programs to help you to keep your skills up to date

Down

1. A form to be filled out when applying for a job

2. To perform your duties properly and to use the correct forms to record client care and billable time

3. The process of judging an employee's performance to determine suitability to remain on the job

5. Wages earned

7. Required

9. Informal method of exchanging information about job openings

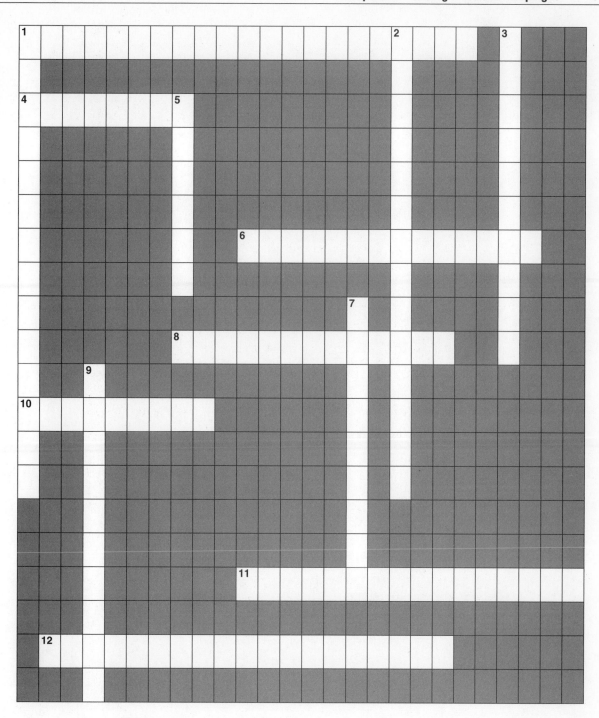

Answers

CHAPTER 1 LEARNING ABOUT HOME CARE

Matching
1. G
2. C
3. D
4. H
5. B
6. E
7. A
8. F

Situations

Situation 1
Response:

Length of course: This answer will be different for each program. Check with your teacher to make sure that you have the correct answer for your training program.

Clinical experience: Learning in the home of a client under the supervision of the instructor or home care nurse.

Evaluation: Judging performance to determine progress in learning.

Situation 2
Response:

I want to do everything that I can do to learn. These are tools to help me do that job.

Situation 3
Response:

Suggest that your classmates tell the teacher what they don't understand. You go to the teacher and tell him or her that you didn't understand certain words and that you need some help.

Practicing to Take Tests
True or False
1. F Home care aide training programs vary in length from state to state.
2. T
3. T
4. F The process of evaluating the home care aide student's performance goes on throughout the entire program.
5. F The client and the family help the instructor to evaluate the student's performance.
6. T

Multiple Choice
1. b
2. c
3. a

Real-Life Situations
Each person will have different answers and different schedules. Be prepared to discuss these in class.

CHAPTER 2 THE HOME CARE INDUSTRY

Matching
1. F
2. J
3. B
4. I
5. C
6. G
7. D
8. K
9. H
10. E
11. L
12. A
13. M

Hidden Words: Qualities of a Home Care Aide

C	E	V	I	T	A	R	E	P	O	O	C	E	P
O	O	E	T	R	E	L	A	P	R	I	O	N	L
M	P	N	L	O	W	I	L	T	T	L	U	T	E
P	A	R	S	B	G	E	N	S	S	U	T	S	A
E	T	L	T	I	A	E	A	C	E	F	N	U	S
T	I	A	B	S	D	I	H	C	N	T	A	O	L
E	E	E	A	I	S	E	L	L	O	C	V	E	U
N	N	N	F	U	E	R	R	E	H	E	R	T	F
T	T	N	H	R	A	K	L	A	R	P	E	R	L
L	O	T	F	E	S	D	I	N	T	S	S	U	L
C	N	U	W	I	L	L	I	N	G	E	B	O	I
E	L	B	A	D	N	E	P	E	D	R	O	C	K
S	I	N	C	E	R	E	G	N	I	R	A	C	S

Word Completion

1. Teaches the client helpful ways to improve swallowing	Speech-language therapist
2. Coordinates the activities of the team	Case manager
3. Supervises the activities of the LPN/LVN and the home care aide	Registered nurse
4. Gives spiritual guidance to the client	Clergy
5. Instructs the client and family about preparing meals according to the diet ordered by the doctor	Dietitian
6. Checks the breathing equipment being used by the client	Respiratory therapist
7. Arranges community services to be provided to the client	Social worker
8. Provides complex nursing care to clients with special needs	Nurse specialist
9. Gives personal care to clients and performs light housekeeping duties	Home care aide
10. Assesses the client's ability to perform ADL	Occupational therapist
11. Gives nursing care to clients whose conditions are stable	Licensed practical nurse
12. Teaches exercises to strengthen the client's leg muscles	Physical therapist

True or False

1. T
2. F Never take any of your client's prescription drugs.
3. F The physical therapist is responsible for evaluating his or her client's progress in physical therapy.
4. F When visitors arrive, keep yourself busy elsewhere in the home.
5. T
6. T
7. F It is important (necessary) to maintain healthy eating habits.
8. T
9. F Politely refuse the beer.
10. F You do not agree to work extra hours. Ask the family to contact the agency about the need for more hours of service.

CHAPTER 3 DEVELOPING EFFECTIVE COMMUNICATION SKILLS

True or False

1. F Hearing-impaired persons will understand what you are saying if you do not exaggerate your words.
2. F It is helpful to keep a pad and pencil nearby so that your *hearing-impaired* client can communicate in writing, if necessary.
3. T
4. T
5. T
6. F Always stand *in front of* visually-impaired clients, because their side vision is not good.
7. T
8. F Speak in *a normal* tone of voice to make sure that your blind client understands what you are saying.
9. F While your client is asking you a question, be sure to concentrate on *what he or she is saying and not on* how you will answer him or her.
10. T
11. T
12. F The client *does not have* the right to refuse care given by an African-American home care aide.
13. F You should *not* compliment her on how attractive she looks to make her feel better.
14. T
15. T

Situations

Situation 1
Response:
"Mr. Walker, you wanted to talk about your wife's illness. Let's go into the living room. What did you want to tell me?"

Action:
Do not go into the bedroom. Report this incident to your supervisor, and prepare a written report.

Situation 2
Response:
"I don't understand, Mr. D'Orio. What do you mean when you say that your son doesn't love you anymore?"

Action:
Document what you have observed and what Mr. D'Orio has said. Report these observations to your supervisor.

Situation 3
Response:
"I think that you need more help than I can give to you, so I'm notifying my supervisor immediately."

Action:
Go and call your supervisor.

Situation 4
Response:
"It's very nice of you to think of me, but I'm not allowed to accept anything from my clients or their families."

Action:
Do not accept the money.

Matching
1. G
2. I
3. A
4. D
5. B
6. K
7. F
8. J
9. C
10. H
11. E

Diagram (Workbook Figure 3-1)

1. Message
2. Meaning
3. Sender
4. Receiver
5. Feedback

Completion

1. Effective communication begins with one basic principle: <u>respect for the client and family as human beings.</u>
2. Five ways to improve listening skills are:
   a. <u>Be quiet.</u>
   b. <u>Stop all other activities.</u>
   c. <u>Listen to the entire message.</u>
   d. <u>Do not interrupt the speaker.</u>
   e. <u>Let the speaker finish.</u>
      Other possible answers:
      Don't think of an answer while another person is speaking.
      Keep confidences.
      Practice listening skills.
3. Two topics to avoid when communicating with your client are <u>religion</u> and <u>politics</u>.
   Other possible answer:
   your personal affairs
4. Confidential information is shared with your supervisor when <u>it is necessary for the care, health, or well-being of client.</u>
5. To be a good listener, you must devote <u>your full attention</u> to the speaker.

CHAPTER 4 UNDERSTANDING YOUR CLIENT'S NEEDS

Diagram (Workbook Figure 4-1)

1. Physical (physiological)
2. Security and safety
3. Love
4. Self-esteem
5. Self-actualization

Completion

1. Oxygen and food are examples of <u>physiological</u> needs.
2. Preventing falls helps to meet a client's need for <u>safety</u>.
3. Feeling close to other persons helps to meet the need for <u>love</u>.
4. Feeling good about one's self is meeting the need for <u>self-esteem</u>.
5. By learning and creating, people meet their need for <u>self-actualization</u>.

True or False

1. <u>T</u>
2. <u>F</u> Families can include grandparents, grandchildren, stepchildren, stepparents, and others.
3. <u>T</u>
4. <u>T</u>
5. <u>T</u>
6. <u>F</u> Family members do not always work together to meet their own needs.
7. <u>F</u> The home care aide cannot meet all of the needs of the client and his or her family.
8. <u>T</u>
9. <u>F</u> Everyone has personal needs.
10. <u>T</u>

Growth and Development

1. Many factors influence growth and development.
2. Early life experiences guide the foundation for our growth and development in later years.
3. Growth occurs in a logical pattern.
4. One stage of growth and development must be completed before moving on to the next stage.
5. Physical growth is completed around the age of 21, but emotional, social, and intellectual growth continue throughout life.

Growth and Development Chart

GROWTH AND DEVELOPMENT CHART (Answers may vary—these are sample suggested answers.)

Development Stage	Age	Characteristics	Ways to Meet Client Needs
Infancy	Birth to 1 year	1. Tremendous growth	1. Hold and cuddle
		2. Learns to control head	2. Provide safe environment
		3. Learns to sit	3. Create dependable, loving, secure world
		4. Says first word	
		5. Begins to walk	
Toddler	1–3 years	1. Endless activity	1. Eliminate hazards
		2. Gets into everything; accident prone	2. Praise safe behavior
		3. Temper tantrums	3. Support parental toilet training program
		4. Plays alone	
Preschool	3–5 years	1. Endless energy	1. Avoid use of "don't"
		2. Eager to learn	2. Provide safe environment
		3. Imaginary playmates	3. Follow rituals for nap time, bed time, meals
		4. Rituals important	
School age	6–12 years	1. Slow, steady growth	1. Follow rules established in home
		2. Active, strong	2. Ensure adequate nutrition
		3. Enjoys friends	3. Respect privacy
		4. Likes challenges	4. Be honest
Adolescent	12–18 years	1. Rapid physical growth	1. Respect privacy
		2. Sexual maturation	2. Follow rules of home
		3. Striving for independence	3. Expect acceptable behavior
		4. Peers important	

Development Stage	Age	Characteristics	Ways to Meet Client Needs
Adulthood	18–65 years	1. Physical development completed	1. Maintain activities of daily living
		2. Career and financial independence	2. Offer choices in routine
		3. Parenting, bonding with partner	3. Involve in family life
Older adulthood	65–100+ years	1. Adjusting to physical changes	1. Provide safety
		2. Adjusting to retirement	2. Encourage independence
		3. Adjusting to death of partner	3. Allow time. Be calm and patient

CHAPTER 5 UNDERSTANDING HOW THE BODY WORKS

Organ	System		Organ	System
1. Pituitary gland	Endocrine		8. Gallbladder	Digestive
2. Liver	Digestive		9. Capillaries	Circulatory
3. Prostate gland	Male reproductive		10. Ovaries	Female reproductive or endocrine
4. Bronchioles	Respiratory		11. Urethra	Urinary
5. Diaphragm	Muscular or respiratory		12. Spinal cord	Nervous
6. Ribs	Skeletal		13. Larynx	Respiratory
7. Arteries	Circulatory		14. Brain	Nervous

Fill in the Blanks

Body System	Function
1. Skeletal	Provides support, protection, and movement
2. Muscular	Allows for movement
3. Circulatory and lymphatic	Transports blood and tissue fluid throughout the body; fights infection
4. Integumentary	Protects the body from injury
5. Nervous	Sends and receives electrical messages; coordinates all body functions
6. Respiratory	Takes in air and removes carbon dioxide from the body
7. Endocrine	Produces hormones that regulate body functions
8. Digestive	Responsible for nutrition and the elimination of body waste
9. Urinary	Filters all the blood to remove dissolved waste and excess water
10. Reproductive	Responsible for the production of offspring

Matching

1. I	6. J
2. D	7. C
3. E	8. B
4. H	9. F
5. G	10. A

Completion

1. Tissues are made up of groups of <u>cells</u>.
2. Another word for *throat* is <u>pharynx</u>.
3. Arteries carry blood <u>from or away from</u> the heart.
4. <u>Capillaries</u> connect arteries to veins.
5. A heart beat has two parts: <u>contraction (systole)</u> and <u>relaxation (diastole)</u>.
6. A body system is made up of many <u>organs</u>.
7. Another word for *windpipe* is <u>trachea</u>.
8. The lid that prevents food from entering the respiratory system is the <u>epiglottis</u>.
9. The long, strong muscles are in the <u>legs</u>.
10. The urethra has two functions in the man because it carries both <u>urine</u> and <u>sperm</u>.

Diagram

Workbook Figure 5-1 (Circulatory System)

1. heart
2. veins
3. arteries

Diagram, cont'd

Workbook Figure 5-2 (Respiratory System)

1. nose
2. pharynx
3. larynx
4. trachea
5. bronchus
6. lungs
7. alveoli

Workbook Figure 5-3 (Digestive System)

1. mouth
2. pharynx
3. esophagus
4. stomach
5. small intestine
6. large intestine
7. liver
8. gallbladder
9. appendix
10. anus

CHAPTER 6 OBSERVING, REPORTING, AND RECORDING

Matching

1. J
2. E
3. L
4. B
5. A
6. I
7. K
8. D
9. F
10. C
11. G
12. H

Reporting and Recording

1. Bruise on client's arm — <u>Record on client's record</u>
2. Client complains of sudden pain in chest — <u>Notify supervisor immediately; record your observations and action taken</u>
3. Foul odor in client's refrigerator — <u>Record your observations and action taken</u>
4. Client having severe difficulty with breathing — <u>Notify supervisor immediately; record your observations and action taken</u>
5. Client has sudden vomiting and diarrhea — <u>Notify supervisor immediately; record your observations and action taken</u>
6. Client's toilet overflowed; client lives alone and has no immediate family nearby — <u>Notify supervisor immediately for directions</u>
7. Client refused lunch and drank one cup of tea — <u>Record your observations; notify supervisor</u>
8. Client cried for half an hour after brother's visit — <u>Record your observations</u>
9. Client's daughter slapped client twice in the face during a 15-minute visit — <u>Record your observations; notify supervisor</u>
10. Client had been irritable but now is pleasant and talkative — <u>Record your observations</u>

True or False

1. T
2. F Care records are confidential and may not be shared with family members.
3. F Only a small portion of the record is in the home; most of it is at the office of the home care agency.
4. T
5. T
6. T
7. F It is not the role of the home care aide to change client care plans.
8. T
9. T
10. F Call your supervisor whenever you feel it is necessary. It is always better to be safe than sorry.

Abbreviations

1. abd — Abdomen/abdominal
2. ADL — Activities of daily living
3. BP — Blood pressure
4. CA — Cancer
5. meds — Medication(s)
6. O_2 — Oxygen
7. OOB — Out of bed
8. ROM — Range of motion
9. Tbsp — Tablespoon
10. TPR — Temperature, pulse, and respirations
11. $\bar{c}$ — With
12. mL — Milliliter
13. $\bar{s}$ — Without
14. tsp — Teaspoon

Recording (Workbook Figure 6-1)

See the "Weekly Client Care Record—Change in Condition" section on p. 23.

WEEKLY CLIENT CARE RECORD—CHANGE IN CONDITION

Date	Time	Observation	Action Taken
00/00/00	9:15 am	Client vomited breakfast. Feels dizzy. Skin blue. Breathing is noisy.	Called supervisor. Called 9-1-1 and client's sister. Ambulance took client and sister to hospital at 9:45 am. Mrs. Jones, supervisor came to home.

Signed: Your name, HCA

Checklist (Workbook Figure 6-1)

WEEKLY CLIENT CARE RECORD

Client _Henry Watkins_   Employee _your name_

Address _123 Harmony Lane_   Title _Home Care Aide_

City _Any town_   State _WV_ Zip _78412_   Client or Account # _62-4813_

Phone (day) _123-456-7890_ (eve.) _____   Week Ending ___6__ / __8__ / __00__

Fill in the date for each day.

Write your initials in the box which corresponds to each task performed.

	DATE	6/2	6/3	6/4	6/5	6/6	6/7	6/8
	DAY	Mon.	Tue.	Wed.	Th.	Fri.	Sat.	Sun.
	TIME ARRIVED	9am						
PERSONAL CARE:								
Bath ☐ Bed ☐ Chair ☑ Shower ☐ Tub		yn						
Perineal Care								
Hair ☐ Groom ☐ Shampoo								
Mouthcare ☐ Denture Care								
Shave								
Nail Care ☐ Clean ☐ File								
Foot Care								
Special Skin Care								
Dressing ☑ Assist ☐ Complete		yn						
Toileting ☐ Bed Pan ☐ Commode ☐ BRP								
Other instructions: _____								
CLIENT ACTIVITIES: Transfer Activity Instructions: _OOB to Chair_		yn						
Assist with walking ☐ Cane ☐ Walker ☐ Crutches								
Assist with exercises ☐ ROM ☐ Other (specify)								
Wheelchair activities								
Other instructions: _____								
OTHER FUNCTIONS:								
Temp. ☐ Oral ☐ Rectal ☐ Underarm ☐ Ear								
Pulse								
Respirations								
Blood Pressure								
Weigh Client		yn						
Record Intake/Output (use special form)								

	Mon.	Tue.	Wed.	Th.	Fri.	Sat.	Sun.
OTHER FUNCTIONS:							
Prepare and serve meal/snack							
Special diet (Specify)							
Assist with feeding							
Medications reminder							
Stoma care							
Incontinent care							
Record bowel movements							
Change in condition (office was notified)							
Other instructions: _____							
HOUSEHOLD SERVICES:							
Change/make client's bed	yn						
Clean client's room							
Clean bathroom	yn						
Clean kitchen; wash dishes							
Vacuum, sweep, dust							
Client laundry	yn						
Marketing							
Errands (specify) _____							
Other instructions: _____							
DEPARTURE TIME	11am						
TOTAL HOURS	2hr						

I certify that the hours shown represent my true total hours worked.

Signature *your name*   Title *Home Care Aide*   Date *6/2/00*

Return form to Home Care Agency weekly.
Notify Home Care Agency if your client's condition has changed since your last visit.

Situation

1. Observe: Find out about the indigestion. What does it feel like?
2. Report: Call your supervisor.
3. Record: Record the client's indigestion, your call to the supervisor, and your actions.

Incident Report (Workbook Figure 6-2)

ABC Home Care Agency
INCIDENT REPORT

PERSON INVOLVED	(Last name)	(First name)	(Middle initial)						
Address	Your name/HCA			Adult ☒ Child ☐	Male ☐ Female ☐		Age Your age		

Date of incident/accident 0/0/00 | Time of incident/accident 10 A.M. ☒ P.M. ☐ | Exact location of incident/accident — Bedroom ☐ Hallway ☐ Bathroom ☐ Other ☒ Specify client's porch

CLIENT ☐ List diagnosis if contributed to incident/accident: DNA

Client's condition before incident/accident
Normal ☐ Confused ☐ Disoriented ☐ Sedated ☐ (Drug _____ Dose _____ Time _____) Other ☐ Specify _____

Were bed rails ordered? Yes ☐ No ☐ | Were bed rails present? Yes ☐ No ☐ | If Yes, Up ☐ Down ☐ | Was height of bed adjustable? Yes ☐ No ☐ | If Yes, Up ☐ Down ☐

EMPLOYEE ☒ | Name Your name/HCA | Job title HCA | Length of time in this position 1 year

VISITOR ☐ OTHER ☐ | Home address Your address | Home phone Your phone number

Occupation HCA | Reason for presence assigned to care for client

Equipment involved ☐ Property involved ☐ Describe DNA | Was person authorized to be at location of incident/accident? Yes ☒ No ☐

Describe exactly what happened; why it happened; what the causes were. If injury, state part of body injured. If property of equipment damaged, describe damage.

My left foot went through weak board on client's porch. Fell and scraped left leg and hurt ankle. Ankle became swollen and sore

Indicate on diagram location of injury:

Temp. _____ Pulse. _____ Resp. _____

B.P. _____

TYPE OF INJURY

1. Laceration ☐
2. Hematoma ☐
3. Abrasion ☒
4. Burn ☐
5. Swelling ☒
6. None apparent ☐
7. Other (specify below) ☐

LEVEL OF CONSCIOUSNESS

_____

Name of supervisor notified Supervisor's name | Time of notification 10:10 A.M./P.M. | Time of responded 10:10 A.M./P.M.

Name and relationship of family member notified DNA | Time of notification _____ A.M./P.M. | Time of responded _____ A.M./P.M.

Was person involved seen by a physician? Yes ☒ No ☐ If Yes, physician's name | Where Medical center | Date 0/0/00 | Time 11:30 A.M. ☒ P.M. ☐

Was first aid administered? Yes ☐ No ☐ If Yes, type of provided by whom | Where | Date | Time A.M. ☐ P.M. ☐

Was person involved taken to a hospital? Yes ☒ No ☐ If Yes, hospital name Medical center | By whom Supervisor | Date 0/0/00 | Time 11:45 A.M. ☒ P.M. ☐

Name, title (if applicable), address & phone no. of witness(es) | Additional comments and/or steps taken to prevent recurrence:

SIGNATURE/TITLE/DATE	**SIGNATURE/TITLE/DATE**
Person preparing report Your name/HCA 0/0/00	Case Manager
Supervisor Supervisor Signature 0/0/00	Administrator

INCIDENT REPORT

CHAPTER 7 WORKING WITH ILL AND DISABLED CLIENTS

Client Reactions

1. A. Anger or frustration
   B. Pick up the fork and say, "This has been a trying day for you. How can I help?"
2. A. Withdrawal
   B. Ignore the behavior. Continue to prepare for her bed bath and talk to her, even if she does not respond.
3. A. Anxiety or fear
   B. Encourage her to do the exercises. Reassure her that you are there to support her so that she will not fall. Demonstrate what you would do if she begins to lose her balance.
4. A. Overdependence
   B. Tell him that he needs to use his arm muscles for good circulation and to grow strong again. Washing his own face is an easy way to begin.
5. A. Denial
   B. Notify your supervisor immediately.

Family Situations

1. *Tucker family*: Listen to Mrs. Tucker. Explain that Mr. Tucker is angry about his illness (rather than angry at her). Assure Mrs. Tucker that her feelings are normal and that others feel this way, too. Notify your supervisor of this conversation, and tell your supervisor what you have already said. Seek further advice. A caregiver support group might be helpful for Mrs. Tucker.
2. *Ann Marie Burroughs*: Listen carefully to what Ann Marie's mother is telling you. Tell the mother that you cannot provide the kind of assistance that might help Anne Marie and that you will call your supervisor for assistance. Call your supervisor, and report what is happening.
3. *Santiago family*: Listen to Jose. Tell him that you will speak with your supervisor about his concerns. The agency will be able to refer him to people who can help him during this difficult period.

Crossword Puzzle

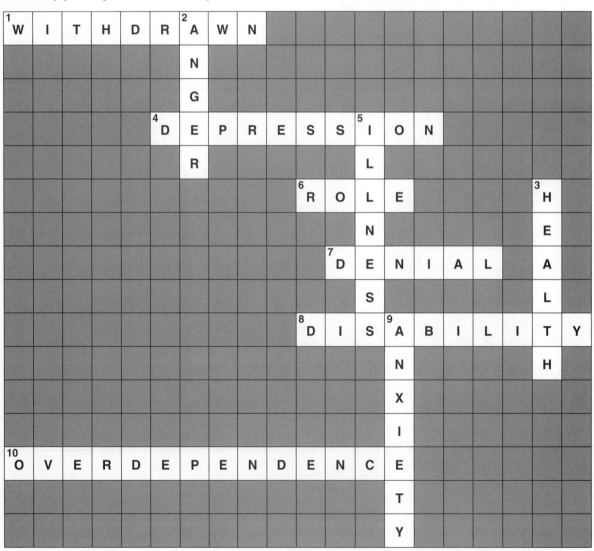

CHAPTER 8 MAINTAINING A SAFE ENVIRONMENT

Home Hazards (Workbook Figure 8-1)

1. Open cabinet door	1. Close the door.
2. Spill on the floor	2. Wipe up the spill.
3. Magazines/newspapers on the floor	3. Pick up the magazines/newspapers
4. Dangling appliance cord	4. Place the cord out of the way.
5. Pot holder next to working gas burner on stove	5. Remove the pot holder.
6. Toys on the floor	6. Pick up the toys.
7. Aerosol can near an open flame	7. Remove the can from the area, and store it properly.
8. Food and cleaning supplies kept together	8. Separate these items, and store them properly.
9. Poisons within reach of children	9. Store these properly.
10. Knives within reach of children	10. Store these properly.

(Other appropriate answers are also acceptable.)

Diagram (Workbook Figure 8-2)

1. Ingredient: Fuel
   Examples may include rubbish, oily rags, clothing, linens, towels, pot holders, paints, paint thinners, alcohol, and perfumes.
2. Ingredient: Oxygen
   Examples may include air and medical oxygen.
3. Ingredient: Heat source
   Examples may include matches, cigarette lighters, pilot lights, faulty plugs and electrical wires, hair dryers, irons, curling irons, burning candles, lit cigarettes, cigars, and pipes.

Matching

1. A and/or C (when lit and burning)
2. C
3. A
4. B
5. C
6. B
7. B
8. A
9. B
10. C
11. A
12. A

Situations

Situation 1

A. Personal safety rules:
   1. Be aware of her surroundings.
   2. Walk confidently, like she knows where she is going.
   3. Carry a whistle, personal alarm, or cellular telephone.
   Other options:
   • *Use well-lighted bus stop that is used often.*
   • *Plan the shortest, safest route possible.*
   • *Do not walk near doorways.*
   • *Have exact change or a token for the bus in her pocket.*
   • *Walk near others.*
   • *Be sure that her wallet or purse is not visible.*
B. Safety rules when riding a bus:
   1. Sit near the bus driver.
   2. If she feels unsafe about getting off at her stop, ride to the next stop.
   3. Do not talk to strangers.

Other options:
   • *Be observant.*
C. Safety rules before reaching the door of the client's apartment or her own home:
   1. Have the house key in her hand.
   2. Don't go inside if she suspects that something is wrong.
   3. Be aware of what is going on around her.
   Other options:
   • *Do not enter the elevator if she suspects that anything is wrong; wait for the next elevator.*

Situation 2

A. Safety rules to follow when traveling to and from client's home:
   1. Keep her doors locked at all times.
   2. Always wear a seatbelt.
   3. Make sure that she has at least half a tank of gas.
   4. Never pick up hitchhikers.

5. Select the most direct route.
6. Let her family know her route.
7. Let the agency know when she leaves home and when she arrives at the client's home (according to agency policy); carry her cellular telephone.
8. Keep her car in good repair.
   Other options:
   • *If the car breaks down, do not get out; put on flashers*

• *If police arrive in an unmarked car, ask for identification before opening the window or door.*
• *Place a "Call Police" placard or sign in the window, and wait for the police to arrive.*
• *Do not the leave car; stay in the locked car, and wait for the police.*
• *Keep her purse or wallet out of sight.*

Situation 3

Yes	Blanket		Yes	Essential medications in childproof containers
Yes	Eating utensils		Yes	Sweater
No	Pots and pans		Yes	Canned food and can opener
Yes	Money, including coins		No	Bottle of liquor
Yes	First aid kit		Yes	Bottle of water
Yes	Extra car keys		No	Shampoo
Yes	Flashlight, including batteries		No	Hairspray
Yes	Important papers (e.g., insurance policies, wills)			

CHAPTER 9 MAINTAINING A HEALTHY ENVIRONMENT

Household Tasks Schedule

Making the client's bed	Daily
Cleaning the refrigerator	Weekly
Cleaning the commode	Daily
Changing the bed linens	Weekly or as needed
Removing trash	Daily
Laundering bed linens	Weekly or as needed
Picking up clutter	Daily
Washing dishes	Daily
Dusting the living room	Weekly
Cleaning the toilet and the bathroom sink	Daily
Sweeping the kitchen floor	Daily
Cleaning the kitchen counters	Daily

Cleaning and Storing Supplies

Dust cloth	Wash in soapy water and air dry
Broom	Shake into large moistened bag and hang
Sponge	Wash in soapy water and air dry
Bucket	Rinse and dry
Toilet brush	Rinse in cold water and store in container
Rubber utility gloves	Rinse exterior and air dry

Sorting Laundry

1. <u>D</u>   Dirty work clothes
2. <u>A</u>   White cotton athletic socks
3. <u>C</u>   Blue toilet lid cover
4. <u>A or C</u> Cotton print sheets
5. <u>E</u>   Nylon underwear
6. <u>A</u>   White cotton sheets
7. <u>B</u>   Blue jeans
8. <u>C</u>   Light purple towels
9. <u>B</u>   Dark brown cotton tee shirt
10. <u>C</u>   Yellow jogging top and pants
11. <u>A</u>   Diapers
12. <u>E</u>   Pink embroidered sweater

True or False

1. <u>F</u> Sick people may be able to care for their own homes.
2. <u>T</u>
3. <u>T</u>
4. <u>T</u>
5. <u>F</u> Never use a sharp knife to remove frost from a freezer.
6. <u>F</u> Do not wash wooden bowls in the automatic dishwasher.
7. <u>T</u>
8. <u>T</u>
9. <u>T</u>
10. <u>T</u>
11. <u>T</u>
12. <u>T</u>

CHAPTER 10 MEETING THE CLIENT'S NUTRITIONAL NEEDS

Fill in the Blank

1. Food energy is measured by means of a unit called a <u>calorie</u>.
2. Carbohydrates are composed of the chemicals <u>carbon</u>, <u>hydrogen</u>, and <u>oxygen</u>.
3. Sugars and starches are examples of <u>carbohydrates</u>.
4. Amino acids are components of <u>proteins</u>.
5. Vitamins A, D, E, and K are <u>fat-soluble</u> vitamins.
6. A tool to use in menu planning is the <u>MyPlate</u> <u>Food Guide</u>.
7. The five groups of the MyPlate Food Guide are <u>grains</u>, <u>vegetables</u>, <u>fruits</u>, <u>dairy</u>, and <u>protein foods</u>.
8. Too much saturated fat may increase the level of <u>cholesterol</u> in the blood.
9. Roughage is another word for <u>fiber</u>.
10. The term that is used to describe poor appetite is <u>anorexia</u>.
11. When assisting a blind client to eat, the plate is described as a <u>clock</u>.
12. Foods high in salt are avoided on a <u>sodium</u>-restricted diet.
13. Spicy, highly seasoned, and fried foods are avoided when following a <u>bland</u> diet.
14. The human body is <u>60</u> percent fluid.
15. The daily need for water (fluids) is at least <u>1 quart or 4 to 6 cups or 1000 to 1500 mL</u>.
16. A lack of fluid in the body can cause <u>dehydration</u>.
17. Three factors to consider during menu planning are <u>food preferences</u>, <u>meal patterns</u>, <u>variety of intake</u>, <u>moderation in intake</u>, <u>balanced diet</u>, and <u>adequate fluids</u>. *(Any three of these are acceptable.)*
18. Butter, cream, and ice cream would be avoided on a <u>low-fat or low-cholesterol</u> diet.
19. Proper storage is essential to preserve the <u>quality</u> and <u>safety</u> of foods.
20. Calcium and phosphorus are examples of <u>minerals</u> found in food and needed by the human body.

Crossword Puzzle

```
                              2
                              M
    1
    B  A  C  T  E  R  I  A
                              L
    3
    P  R  O  T  E  I  N
                              U
                              T
          4                              5
          D  E  H  Y  D  R  A  T  E  D
                              I        E
       7                                 F
       U                      T        I
       N                      I        C
    6                         O
    N  U  T  R  I  T  I  O  N          I
       P                              E
       R                              N
       I                              C
       C                              Y
       E
```

My Plate Food Guide (Workbook Figure 10-1)

1. A. Fruits
   B. Vegetables
   C. Grains
   D. Protein foods
   E. Dairy

2. A. Blueberries
   Orange
   Apples
   (Other fruits are acceptable here as well.)

   B. Spinach
      Carrots
      Kidney beans
      (Other vegetables and legumes are acceptable here as well.)
   C. Whole grain bread
      Cereal
      Rice
      (Other grains are acceptable here as well.)

   D. Chicken
      Fish
      Eggs
      (Other protein foods are acceptable here as well.)
   E. Milk
      Yogurt
      Cottage cheese
      (Other dairy foods are acceptable here as well.)

Matching

1. A, B, C
2. D
3. A
4. A, B, C
5. C
6. A, B, C
7. C

8. A
9. D
10. A
11. D
12. C
13. A, B, C, D

Therapeutic Diets (Workbook Figure 10-2)

The diets described here are not meant to be the only correct answers; rather, they are intended to give you an idea of the changes or substitutions that you will need to make for clients who have diet restrictions.

A	B	C	D
REGULAR	HIGH FIBER	LOW SODIUM	LOW FAT/LOW CHOLESTEROL
Canned or Homemade Soup	Canned or Homemade Pea, Bean, or Vegetable Soup	Low-Sodium Canned or Homemade Soup	Low-Fat Canned or Homemade Soup
Ham Sandwich on Bread	Turkey Sandwich on Whole Wheat Bread	Low-Salt Turkey Sandwich on Bread	Low-Fat Turkey Breast on Reduced-Calorie Bread
Mayonnaise	Mayonnaise or Mustard		Mustard or Low-Fat Mayonnaise
Lettuce and Tomato	Lettuce and Tomato	Lettuce and Tomato	Lettuce and Tomato
Whole Milk	Whole Milk	Low-Fat/Fat-free Milk	Low-Fat/Fat-free Milk
Cookies	Fresh Fruit	Fresh Fruit	Fresh Fruit

Situations

Situation 1

Milk	Amount; type (e.g., fat-free, 1%, 2%, evaporated)
Bread	Amount; type (e.g., white, whole wheat)
Orange juice	Amount; frozen, fresh, or concentrate; pulp, no pulp, added calcium
Eggs	Amount; white or brown
Ground beef	Amount; type (e.g., chuck, round, fat content)
Carrots	Amount; fresh, frozen, or canned
Bananas	Amount; type; size; color
Broccoli	Amount; fresh or frozen
Toilet paper	Amount; color; brand name
Ice cream	Amount, flavor; brand name; type (e.g., fat free, ice milk, frozen yogurt)

Situation 2

Milk	Refrigerator
Bread	Refrigerator or pantry
Orange juice	Refrigerator or freezer
Eggs	Inside the refrigerator (i.e., not in the refrigerator door)
Ground beef	Refrigerator for immediate use, otherwise the freezer
Carrots	Refrigerator
Bananas	Pantry
Broccoli	Refrigerator or freezer
Toilet paper	Bathroom closet or pantry
Ice cream	Freezer

Situation 3

Response: Tell Mrs. Smith that you cannot take her any-where without following the agency's rules.
Action: Notify your supervisor.

CHAPTER 11 PREVENTING INFECTION/MEDICAL ASEPSIS

Matching

1. F
2. G
3. C
4. K
5. A
6. D
7. I
8. L
9. B
10. H
11. E
12. J

True or False

1. T
2. F Standard (universal) precautions are used for all clients.
3. F When in doubt about disinfecting items in the home, ask your supervisor.
4. T
5. F Microorganisms are found everywhere.
6. T
7. F OSHA regulations concerning bloodborne pathogens must be followed by anyone who may come in contact with blood or other body fluids.
8. T
9. T
10. T

Completion
1. To grow and multiply, all microorganisms need <u>moisture</u>, <u>warmth</u>, and <u>food</u>; or <u>host</u>, <u>darkness</u>, and <u>oxygen</u>.
2. Boil items for <u>20</u> minutes to destroy pathogenic organisms.
3. When preparing vinegar solution, use <u>one</u> part vinegar to <u>three</u> parts water.
4. Disinfection using the oven requires that items be baked for <u>1 hour</u> at a temperature of <u>350°</u> F (<u>180°</u> C).
5. When preparing bleach solution, use <u>one</u> part bleach to <u>ten</u> parts water.
6. Bleach solution must be put in a plastic container. The label must contain this information: <u>name of solution (bleach)</u>, <u>strength (1:10)</u>, <u>date</u>, and <u>time</u>.
7. Handwashing is required <u>before</u> and <u>after</u> giving client care.
8. The most common household disinfecting solution is <u>soap</u> or <u>detergent</u> and <u>hot water</u>.
9. Microorganisms can be transmitted by means of <u>food</u>, <u>water</u>, <u>insects</u>, <u>direct</u> or <u>indirect</u> human contact, <u>animals</u>, and <u>air</u>.
10. Factors that help to increase the risk for infectious diseases include:
    a. <u>Age</u>
    b. <u>Great stress</u>
    c. <u>Poor living conditions</u>
    d. <u>Chronic or acute illness</u>
    e. <u>Poor nutrition</u>

Situations
1. Wash your hands.
   Cleanse the wound with antiseptic.
   Notify your supervisor immediately.
2. Remove the can and discard it.
   Wash your hands.
   Give him a box of tissues. Teach him to cough into the tissue and then to discard the tissue into a plastic bag.
   Discuss the situation with your supervisor.
3. Discard them in a plastic milk jug.
   Discard them in a coffee can.
   Discard them in accordance with agency or community policy.

4. The protective equipment that you would use:
   <u>Gloves and a plastic apron</u>
   How you would transport the soiled clothing and linen to the laundry area in the basement of the home:
   <u>In a plastic bag</u>
   How you would pretreat and launder the soiled linens:
   <u>While wearing gloves, remove and wash away any solid material with cold water. Rinse the linens, and then wash them in hot water with detergent and bleach.</u>

Cycle of Infection (Workbook Figure 11-1)
1. Pathogenic organism
2. Reservoir
3. Exit from reservoir
4. Method of transmission
5. Entrance into a new host
6. Host

CHAPTER 12 BODY MECHANICS

Procedures
1. Applying a transfer (gait) belt:
   <u>4</u>
   <u>5</u>
   <u>1</u>
   <u>2</u>
   <u>3</u>
   <u>6</u>

2. Standing transfer from bed to chair/wheelchair:
   <u>3</u>
   <u>1</u>
   <u>4</u>
   <u>6</u>
   <u>2</u>
   <u>5</u>

3. Assist the client to sit on the side of the bed:
   <u>2</u>
   <u>6</u>
   <u>3</u>
   <u>4</u>
   <u>5</u>
   <u>1</u>

4. Raising the client's head and shoulders:

<u>1</u>

<u>4</u>

<u>6</u>

<u>2</u>

<u>3</u>

<u>5</u>

5. Moving the client to the side of the bed:

<u>1</u>

<u>4</u>

<u>5</u>

<u>3</u>

<u>6</u>

<u>2</u>

Identify the Incorrect Posture

1. Figure 12-1: Bend at the knees to pick up the box.
2. Figure 12-2: Stand up straight with the shoulders back. Pull in the stomach muscles.
3. Figure 12-3: Move the walker closer to the body so that all legs are on the floor. Encourage the client to stand erect, to wear sturdy shoes, and to belt the robe.

Matching

1. E
2. I
3. D
4. J
5. B
6. A
7. H
8. C
9. G
10. F

Situations

1. Explain that there is an easier and safer way to get out of bed. Demonstrate the procedure.
2. Make her comfortable on the floor. Call your supervisor immediately.

Identify the Position

1. Prone
2. Sims'
3. Lateral or side-lying
4. Supine
5. Fowler's

Safety Factors

1. Use a wide base of support.
2. Wear flat or low-heeled shoes.
3. Use the long muscles of the arms and legs.
4. Keep the back straight.
5. Have a plan of action.
6. Lock the brakes on the bed and the wheelchair.
7. Adjust the bed to a convenient working height (or kneel or squat).
8. Have the client help as much as possible so that you don't have to do all the work.
9. Have the client wear shoes.
10. Use a transfer belt to help with the process.

CHAPTER 13 BEDMAKING

Diagram (Workbook Figure 13-1)

A. Blanket

B. Drawsheet

C. Pillowcase

D. Top sheet

E. Bottom sheet

True or False

1. <u>T</u>
2. <u>T</u>
3. <u>T</u>
4. <u>T</u>
5. <u>F</u> Do not use a dry cleaner's bag, because it can be harmful to the client.
6. <u>F</u> An occupied bed is made while the client remains in bed.
7. <u>T</u>
8. <u>T</u>
9. <u>F</u> Do not shake the linens at any time.
10. <u>T</u>
11. <u>F</u> Hold the linens away from your clothing.
12. <u>T</u>
13. <u>T</u>
14. <u>F</u> The most important reason for making a clean, neat, wrinkle-free bed is for the client's comfort.
15. <u>F</u> Do not wash the egg-crate foam mattress pad, because washing will remove the fireproofing. Instead, discard the soiled pad, and then replace it.

CHAPTER 14 PERSONAL CARE

Procedures

1. Giving a back rub:

   6
   3
   2
   4
   5
   1

2. Giving a complete bed bath:

   5
   4
   6
   3
   1
   2

3. Giving a shower in the bathtub:

   4
   5
   6
   2
   3
   1

4. Shaving a male client with a blade razor:

   1
   3
   4
   6
   5
   2

5. Caring for the client's hair:

   4
   1
   2
   3
   6
   5

6. Caring for the client's dentures:

   3
   2
   4
   6
   5
   1

True or False

1. F Personal care is given in accordance with the care plan.
2. T
3. F Dentures are cleaned with warm water and toothpaste.
4. T
5. T
6. T
7. F The chair used should have suction cups at the base of its legs.
8. T
9. T
10. T
11. F Weights are not used, and deep knee bends are not done. Instead, the joints are taken through the normal range of motion.
12. T
13. F Encourage clients to perform as much self-care as possible.
14. T
15. T

What Needs To Be Corrected

1. A. The aide is not wearing gloves. There is no towel across the client's chest. The aide's hand should not be on the client's head.
   B. The aide must wear gloves. Place a towel across the client's chest. Remove the aide's hand from client's head.
2. A. The client's dentures, hearing aids, and eyeglasses are not properly stored. The urinal should not be on the bedside stand.
   B. Put the dentures in a cup with a lid; put the hearing aids in a proper storage container; put the eyeglasses in a case, and place the case in a drawer. The urinal needs to be emptied and not placed near a drinking glass; the urinal should then be stored properly.
3. A. The bedpan should not be on the floor.
   B. The bedpan should be stored out of sight.
4. A. Bed linens should not be placed on the floor.
   B. Place the bed linens in a laundry basket.
5. A. The side rails are down.
   B. When the client is in bed with the bed at the highest level, the side rails should be up.

CHAPTER 15 ELIMINATION

Procedures

1. Giving and removing a bedpan:

   3
   4
   1
   5
   2
   6

2. Giving and removing a urinal:

   2
   6
   4
   3
   1
   5

3. Caring for a client with an indwelling catheter:

   6
   1
   4
   2
   5
   3

4. Applying a condom catheter:

   1
   5
   3
   6
   2
   4

What Needs To Be Corrected?

1. A. The Foley bag is above the bladder. (*Extra credit:* The client has bare feet.)
   B. Lower the bag. (*Extra credit:* Put shoes on the client's feet.)

2. A. The catheter tubing is dangling, and the collection bag is on the side rail.
   B. Properly pin the tubing to the bottom sheet, and position the bag on the bed frame.

3. A. The client is wearing a leg bag in bed.
   B. Remove the leg bag. Connect the client to a regular drainage bag and tubing.

4. A. The collection bag is hanging on the wrong side of the side rail.
   B. Move the collection bag so that it hangs freely behind the side rail and on the bed frame.

5. A. The catheter tubing is kinked, and the bag is on the outside of the bed rail.
   B. Straighten the tubing, and make sure that it is properly pinned to the bottom sheet. Position the collection bag properly.

Situations

1. I = <u>600</u> mL

   O = <u>375</u> mL and <u>one small bowel movement</u>.

2. *Any of the following are acceptable answers for A, B, and C:*

   Know the client's bowel habits, and assist her to the commode immediately.

   Encourage the client to drink water and other fluids and to eat high-fiber foods.

   Do not make the client wait when she has an urge to have a bowel movement.

   Provide privacy for the client.

3. A. Notify your supervisor about the situation.
   B. Clean the client's skin with soap and warm water. Rinse and dry the skin thoroughly.

4. A. Tell the companion that you will notify your supervisor.
   B. 1. Provide skin care to the client.
      2. Dispose of fecal matter from the pouch.
      3. Clean the pouch.

Completion

1. Three characteristics of normal urine are <u>light yellow</u>, <u>clear</u>, and <u>slightly acid odor</u>.

2. Two characteristics of a normal bowel movement are <u>light to dark brown</u> and <u>semisolid</u>.

3. The medical term that is used to describe air or gas in the intestine that is passed through the rectum is *flatus*.

4. Two kinds of gas-forming foods are <u>beans</u> and <u>cabbage</u>.

5. When clients are not able to control urination and/or bowel movements, the medical term used to describe this condition is *incontinence*.

6. If you notice changes in your client's urine or bowel movements, notify your <u>supervisor</u>.

7. Your client has not had a bowel movement for more than 1 week, and he complains of abdominal discomfort. In addition, you notice that small amounts of fecal liquid have leaked from the client's anus. These may be signs that your client has a <u>fecal impaction</u>.

8. Waste materials are eliminated from the body by <u>perspiration from the skin</u>, <u>urine</u>, <u>carbon dioxide and moisture from the lungs</u>, and <u>bowel movements</u>.

9. The medical term for material that is eliminated from the large intestine is *feces*.

10. The medical term that is used to describe the process of eliminating solid waste through the anus is *defecation*.

11. When waste products in the large intestine move so rapidly that the water is not able to be absorbed, this is called *diarrhea*.

12. When providing perineal care or removing a bedpan, it is important to <u>wear disposable gloves</u>.

13. Three ways to help clients to maintain normal urination are:
    A. <u>Provide privacy</u>.
    B. <u>Give the client enough time to urinate</u>.
    C. <u>Position the client in a normal voiding position</u>.

CHAPTER 16 COLLECTING SPECIMENS

Procedures

1. Collecting a routine urine specimen:

    <u>3</u>
    <u>1</u>
    <u>6</u>
    <u>2</u>
    <u>4</u>
    <u>5</u>

2. Collecting a stool specimen:

    <u>1</u>
    <u>4</u>
    <u>2</u>
    <u>3</u>
    <u>6</u>
    <u>5</u>

3. Collecting a sputum specimen:

    <u>5</u>
    <u>3</u>
    <u>6</u>
    <u>1</u>
    <u>4</u>
    <u>2</u>

True or False

1. <u>T</u>
2. <u>F</u> Have the client discard used lancets in accordance with agency and community policy.
3. <u>F</u> Label specimen container with the client's name and address as well as the date and time of specimen collection.
4. <u>T</u>
5. <u>T</u>
6. <u>T</u>
7. <u>F</u> Fill the container only 3/4 full.
8. <u>F</u> Always wear gloves when collecting specimens.
9. <u>F</u> Collect 2 tablespoons of stool.
10. <u>F</u> When collecting this particular 24-hour urine specimen, discard the 3 pm Thursday specimen, and then save all urine during the 24-hour period that follows, including the specimen voided at 3 pm on Friday.

Crossword Puzzle

```
  1
  A
  N
  A
2 C L E A N 3C A T C H
  Y       O
  S       N
  I     4 S T O O L
  S       A
          M
          I
          N     5     6           8
          N     C     C           G
        7 L A B O R A T O R Y     L
          A     N     L           O
        9 U R I N E 7 T     L     V
          T     D     C           E
                I     U
                I  10 L A N C E T S
                N     I
                E
             11 P A R A S I T E S
```

What Needs To Be Corrected?

1. A. The label is on the lid rather than on the container.
   B. Place the label on the container.
2. A. The container is too full.
   B. Discard some of the specimen so that the container is 3/4 full.
3. A. No gloves are being worn.
   B. Put gloves on.
4. A. The information on the label is incomplete.
   B. Complete the information that is needed.

CHAPTER 17 MEASURING VITAL SIGNS

Reading the Thermometer (Workbook Figure 17-1, *A* through *F*)

A. 97° F
B. 100.8° F
C. 99.2° F
D. 102.6° F
E. 98.4° F
F. 101.2° F

Reading the Dial of the Blood Pressure Cuff (Workbook Figure 17-2, *A* through *D*)

A. 110/72
B. 126/92
C. 220/94
D. 168/78

Matching

1. J
2. M
3. K
4. L
5. I
6. A
7. N
8. E
9. G
10. F
11. O
12. B
13. D
14. H
15. C

Reporting Vital Signs

1. X
2. _
3. _
4. X
5. X
6. _
7. _
8. X
9. X
10. X
11. _
12. X
13. _
14. _
15. X

Completion

1. Vital signs give important information about the body processes of <u>circulation</u>, <u>breathing</u>, and heat <u>regulation</u>.
2. Take the client's vital signs when the client is <u>resting</u>.
3. Factors that cause vital signs to increase are <u>exercise</u>, <u>age</u>, and <u>illness</u>. *(Other answers may include pain, medications, and fear.)*
4. Heat leaves the body by means of <u>exhaling</u> and <u>urine</u>.
5. It is 9:30 AM, and your client has just had a big cup of hot coffee. You should take the oral temperature at <u>9:45 AM</u>.
6. Have the client hold the thermometer in the mouth for <u>3</u> minutes before you remove and read the thermometer.
7. To read the thermometer, hold it at <u>eye</u> level.
8. Remove the electronic thermometer and read the digital display window when you hear the <u>beep</u>.
9. Read the <u>last</u> dot to change color on the disposable thermometer.
10. Your client has diarrhea. Do not take a <u>rectal</u> temperature.
11. The normal systolic pressure in an adult is <u>under 120</u>. The normal diastolic pressure in an adult is <u>under 80</u>.
12. The normal range of TPRs in adults is:
    T (O): <u>97.6° to 99.6° F (36.5° to 37.5° C)</u>
    P: <u>60 to 100</u>
    R: <u>12 to 20</u>

13. Before and after using the stethoscope, clean the earpieces and the chestpiece to prevent the <u>spread</u> of <u>pathogens</u>.

14. Shake down the oral thermometer to <u>95° F (35° C)</u> before placing it under the client's tongue.

15. When cleaning the rectal thermometer, begin at the <u>stem</u>, and then wipe <u>downward</u> toward the <u>bulb</u>. Use a <u>twisting</u> motion.

16. Do not use your <u>thumb</u> to take your client's pulse.

17. You begin to take your client's pulse at 10:35 AM. You finish taking this pulse at <u>10:36</u> AM. You continue holding the pulse while you count respirations. You finish counting the respirations at <u>10:37</u> AM.

CHAPTER 18 SPECIAL PROCEDURES

Situation

Situation 1

A. Put gauze or cotton balls between the straps and the client's ears.

Apply water-soluble lubricant around the client's nostrils.

Offer the client fluids frequently.

Put water-soluble lubricant on the client's lips.

Provide frequent oral hygiene.

B. Remove matches, lighters, cigarettes, and cigars from the area.

Place a "no smoking" sign in the room where oxygen is being used.

Have an exit plan to follow in case of fire.

Know the location of a fully charged and functional fire extinguisher.

Place a "no smoking" sign on the front door of Olga's home.

Situation 2

A. Red skin

Blisters on the skin

Client complains of burning sensations in the area

Client complains of pain in the area

B. Check the client's skin every 10 minutes. Diabetic patients are at risk for burns.

C. Record what you have observed on the client care record.

Contact your supervisor for further instructions.

Situation 3

A. Explain that, according to state law, you are not permitted to give any medications or injections. Vitamins are considered drugs.

B. Notify your supervisor.

Situation 4

A. Ask Mrs. Choi to tell you more about her leg cramps. Tell her that you must report her symptoms to your supervisor. This way, she may get relief and not have to be uncomfortable.

B. Notify your supervisor immediately.

C. Do not permit the client to take the medication. Notify your supervisor.

Procedures

1. Giving a sitz bath:
   <u>2</u>
   <u>3</u>
   <u>1</u>
   <u>4</u>
   <u>6</u>
   <u>5</u>

2. Applying hot compresses:
   <u>4</u>
   <u>2</u>
   <u>6</u>
   <u>5</u>
   <u>1</u>
   <u>3</u>

3. Applying an elastic stocking:
   <u>3</u>
   <u>1</u>
   <u>6</u>
   <u>5</u>
   <u>2</u>
   <u>4</u>

4. Assisting with transdermal disks:
   <u>2</u>
   <u>6</u>
   <u>5</u>
   <u>4</u>
   <u>3</u>
   <u>1</u>

Matching

1. F
2. G
3. A
4. E
5. B
6. H
7. C
8. I
9. D
10. J

True or False

1. T
2. T
3. F A full glass of water or another cool liquid is recommended.
4. T
5. T
6. T
7. T
8. F Clients should never take a double dose of medication, because they may end up taking too much of the drug (i.e., overdosing). If a dose is omitted, notify your supervisor.
9. F Tell the client not to take the medication until you have spoken with your supervisor.
10. T
11. T
12. F Unused medications should be discarded.
13. F Vaseline is not water soluble. Use a water-soluble lubricant (e.g., K-Y Jelly).
14. T
15. T
16. F Check the client's skin every 10 minutes or more frequently for clients who are at great risk for burns.
17. T
18. F Keeping the legs under hot water causes the blood vessels in the legs to dilate. This decreases circulation to the perineal area.
19. T
20. T
21. F Home care aides NEVER regulate the flow of intravenous fluids. If there is a problem, call your supervisor.
22. T
23. T
24. T
25. F If elastic bandages are too tight, they will shut off circulation. Apply elastic bandages firmly but not too tightly.

What Needs To Be Corrected?

1. Unplug and remove the electric razor. Explain the risk of fire to the client and the family.
2. Use proper body mechanics, and bend at the knees. Elevate the client's leg. Perform the procedure while the client is in bed.
3. Properly tape the dressing (as shown in Figure 18-14 in the text).
4. The bag of frozen peas should be covered.

CHAPTER 19 CARING FOR OLDER ADULTS

True or False

1. F Aging begins at birth.
2. F Incontinence is not a normal part of aging.
3. T
4. F One's personality usually does not change as aging progresses.
5. F Mental confusion is an abnormal condition.
6. F Do not try to change the subject; instead, listen and be patient.
7. F The need for home care will increase because of the increased numbers of older adults.
8. T
9. F The rate of aging depends on many factors, including heredity, lifestyle, stresses in one's life, and one's occupation.
10. T
11. F It may take a little longer, but older adults can learn new things.
12. T
13. F Individuals who are 85 years old and older represent the most rapidly growing age group.
14. F Explain what you are going to do. Older adults understand what you say, and they need to know what will happen.
15. F Only 4.1% of older adults are cared for in institutions.

Normal Conditions of Aging

1. Difficulty adjusting to a dark room
   - Have the client wait a few minutes until the eyes have a chance to adjust to the darkness.
   - Use a night light.
2. Forgetting where eyeglasses were placed
   - Encourage the client to form the habit of always placing the eyeglasses in the same place.
   - Encourage the client to write reminders on a notepad.
3. Dry skin
   - Use soap sparingly.
   - Apply moisturizers to the skin after a bath.

4. Dry mouth
   - Offer fluids frequently, and give 1.5 to 2 qt (1500 to 2000 mL) daily.
   - Provide mouth care more frequently.
5. Feeling cold
   - Help the client to put on an extra sweater or to use an extra blanket.
   - Tell the client not to use a heating pad or a hot water bottle.
6. Occasional constipation
   - Offer fluids frequently.
   - Serve fruits, vegetables, and other high-fiber foods.
7. Shortness of breath with increased activity
   - Provide frequent rest periods while assisting the client with activities of daily living.
8. Feeling anxious about changes in routine
   - Do not change routines, if possible.
9. Having an urgent need to void
   - For women, clothing should be easy to remove.
   - Assist the client to the bathroom at least every 2 hours.
10. Feeling bloated
    - Avoid serving the client gas-forming foods.
    - Offer the client six to eight small meals per day.
11. Rapid heart beat when under stress
    - Allow plenty of time to perform care procedures.
    - Pace activities to avoid rushing.
12. Trouble adjusting to depths (e.g., going up and down stairs)
    - Encourage the client to use hand rails, if available.
    - Provide support.
13. Having trouble understanding what you are saying
    - Speak to the client slowly and clearly.
    - Use short sentences.
14. Thick, hard toenails
    - Do not cut or file the toenails.
    - Notify your supervisor; a podiatrist may be needed.
15. Experiencing unsteadiness when rising suddenly from a chair
    - Have the client count to 10 after rising and before proceeding to walk.
    - Help the client to walk after he or she counts to 10.

Situations

1. A. "You must be very upset. I don't know what I can do to help, but I will talk to my supervisor about what you have told me." Encourage the daughter to contact your supervisor or the case manager.
   B. Leave the cases of beer under the bed.
   C. Notify your supervisor. Record what you said to the daughter, what you found, what you did about the cases of beer, and that you notified the supervisor.
2. A. Use nonverbal communication (e.g., a hug, touching the client's hand) to show your concern.
   B. Report this situation to the supervisor after giving care to Magdalena.
   C. Record what Magdalena's nephew said, information about Magdalena's physical and emotional states, and that the supervisor was called.
   D. "I can understand how upset you and your wife must be. Magdalena appears to be very upset, too. I was disturbed to see that Magdalena was so upset. I will contact my supervisor; perhaps we can find some solution to the problem."
3. A. Notify the supervisor.
   B. Help Mr. Lewis to be properly groomed.
   C. Clean up the kitchen.
   D. Record all of the actions that you performed.

CHAPTER 20 CARING FOR MOTHERS, INFANTS, AND CHILDREN

Matching

1. C
2. E
3. I
4. G
5. J
6. D
7. A
8. F
9. H
10. B

Recognizing Normal and Abnormal Conditions in the Mother

1. _
2. _
3. X
4. _
5. X
6. X
7. X
8. _
9. _
10. X
11. X
12. X
13. _
14. X
15. _
16. X
17. X
18. X
19. _
20. _

Situations

1. A. Put your arm around her and comfort her. Sit with her, and listen to what she tells you. Offer to make her a cup of tea.
   B. Proceed to give her care as indicated in the care plan. Record the care given, what the client said, and that your supervisor was notified. Report this incident to your supervisor.
2. A. Explain that Johnny's behavior is normal. He is jealous of all the attention that the new baby is getting.
   B. Report this to your supervisor.
   C. Help Yolanda to find ways to give Johnny some special attention and to let him know that he is still special to her.

True or False

1. T
2. F Infants sleep most of the day.
3. T
4. F Stools of breast-fed infants are pasty and mustard colored.
5. F Infants are burped halfway through a feeding as well as at the end of the feeding.
6. T
7. T
8. T
9. F Newborns eat every 2 to 4 hours.
10. F Bottles warmed in the microwave may get too hot and burn the baby's mouth or skin. Place the bottle in a pan of warm water.
11. T
12. T
13. F Children feel stress and experience strong reactions.
14. T
15. T

Observation

1. X
2. _
3. _
4. _
5. _
6. _
7. X
8. X
9. _
10. _

CHAPTER 21 CARING FOR CLIENTS WITH
MENTAL ILLNESS

Situations

1. A. Offer finger foods and individual serving containers of fluid, if available, that can be eaten while pacing.
   B. Follow the care plan schedule for toileting.
      Maintain the client's fluid intake by offering fluids frequently.
   C. Assist the client with hygiene and grooming, as needed.

2. Help the client to dress correctly. Give directions in short, simple sentences: "Put on your socks. Put on your shoes. Tie your shoe laces."
   Encourage his wife to obtain an easy-to-read clock and calendar to help inform him about the time and date.
   Place the detergent and other potentially harmful substances and objects out of reach to provide a safe, secure environment.

3. A. Offer foods that cannot be tampered with (e.g., hard-cooked eggs in their shells with no cracks) and individual unopened servings of food.
   B. Listen to what your client tells you. Tell him that you do not see or hear what he is seeing or hearing.
   C. Notify your supervisor immediately. Do not argue with the client.

4. A. Offer finger foods, small sandwiches, pieces of cheese, crackers, and other small foods that are rich in nutrition (e.g., raisins, grapes). Serve the client small, frequent feedings rather than three big meals. Report to your supervisor. Use a straw so that the client doesn't have to lift a glass or cup. Put only a small amount of liquid into the glass. Use very small glasses, but offer drinks frequently.
   B. Take the client to the bathroom according to schedule in the care plan. Have the client use a commode, if appropriate.
   C. Acknowledge the client's feelings by saying, "You seem very unhappy today."
   D. Report the client's comments to your supervisor. He may be considering suicide.

5. A. Watch the client carefully. Try to find some diversions for her such, as playing cards or checkers or reading to her. Attach a bell to the door to serve as a signal when it is opened. Take her out, when possible, to sit on the porch or walk in the neighborhood. Dress the client in layers that take some time to remove.
   B. Keep a large robe handy, wrap it around the client, and redress her without any comment regarding her "good" or "bad" behavior.

6. Notify your supervisor.

7. A. Tell her, "No, thank you. I need to be alert to care for my client. I don't use anything like that."
   B. Notify your supervisor.

Crossword Puzzle

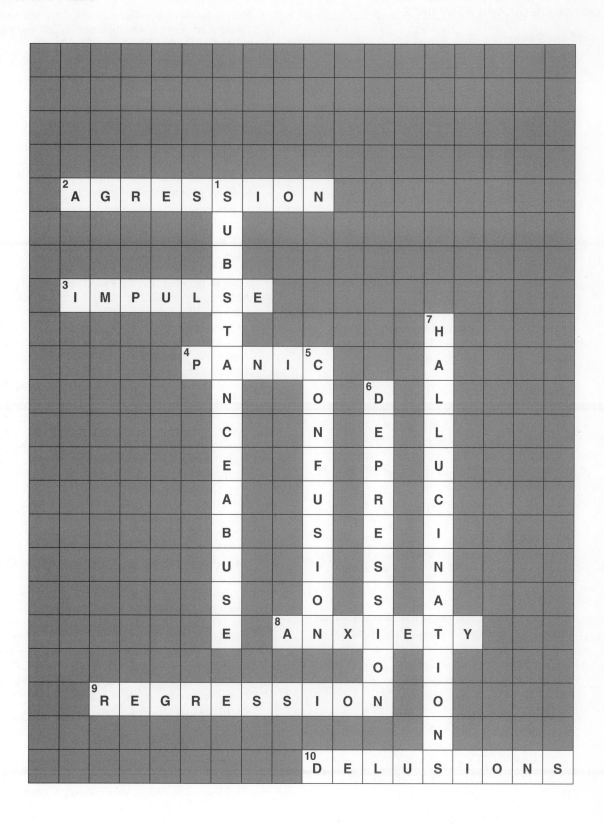

CHAPTER 22 CARING FOR CLIENTS WITH ILLNESSES REQUIRING HOME CARE

Client Conditions

1. Wandering
   - Approach the client calmly and gradually guide him or her back if he or she is wandering outside of the home.
   - Distract the client with an offer of a favorite snack or drink.
   - Make sure that the client wears an identification bracelet.

2. Fatigue
   - Perform care activities when the client's energy is at its highest level, if possible.
   - Allow plenty of time for the client to perform activities of daily living, and do not rush him or her.
   - Provide frequent rest periods for the client during bathing or dressing.

3. Difficulty swallowing
   - Give thickened liquids and pureed or soft foods.
   - Avoid foods that require a lot of chewing.
   - Encourage the client to use techniques that he or she has been taught by the speech-language therapist.

4. Pain
   - Use the techniques listed in the care plan to help the client to tolerate pain (e.g., back rub, the application of heat or cold to the affected area).
   - Bring pain medication to the client on time, in accordance with the care plan.

5. Paralysis or weakness on the right side of the body
   - Do not pull on the right arm or leg when lifting or moving the client.
   - Help the client to use assistive devices (e.g., soap on a rope) as directed by the occupational or physical therapist.

6. Diarrhea
   - Keep the client's anal area clean and dry. Wear disposable gloves when cleaning the client's skin and anal area.
   - Keep a bedpan or commode handy for easy use.
   - Encourage the client to drink lots of fluids, in accordance with the care plan.

7. Difficulty breathing
   - Place the client in Fowler's position, or use two or more pillows to support the upper back.
   - Use energy-saving techniques, such as providing frequent rest periods during bathing and dressing. Do not rush the client.

8. Sores in the mouth
   - Be gentle when providing mouth care, and wear disposable gloves. Use normal saline solution instead of alcohol-based mouthwash.
   - Use a soft-bristled toothbrush or foam swab.

Situations

1. A.1. Lock the doors of any dangerous areas (e.g., basement, garage).
   2. Remove matches, lighter fluid, and other flammable liquids.
   3. Remove the control knobs from the stove.
   4. Place plastic bags out of reach.
   5. Remove food-shaped kitchen magnets, coins, and other small objects.
   B. Try to find the location of Mrs. Gable's favorite hiding places (e.g., under the bed or pillows), and then check these places first. Remain calm, and offer to help her find the eyeglasses.
   C. Make nametags for each family member. Include each person's name and title (e.g., daughter, son-in-law, granddaughter) to help Mrs. Gable to remember. Have the family members wear the nametags. You may wish to make nametags for additional relatives and friends.
   D. Be alert for signs that Mrs. Gable needs to use the bathroom (e.g., restlessness). Plan a routine that involves taking her to the toilet before accidents occur. Put a sign that says "Bathroom" and a picture of a toilet on the bathroom door.
   E. Support groups help caregivers in a variety of ways, including providing the chance to share caregiving experiences with others in similar situations and discussing different ways to handle problems. Susan may find that participating in the support group will give her encouragement and strength to continue to care for her mother.

2. A. Place a chair in the bathroom so that Mr. Yancy can sit by the sink. Place toilet articles within easy reach for Mr. Yancy to use.
   B. Do not wash off the markings, and do not wash the skin inside of the markings.
   C. Select foods that do not require a lot of energy to chew. Offer small, frequent meals. Prepare foods that Mr. Yancy enjoys eating. In addition, prepare foods for consumption (e.g., pour coffee, butter bread) so that Mr. Yancy can use his energy to eat (and not for these activities).
   D. Changes in the type or frequency of pain
      Signs of infection
      Bruising or bleeding
      Problems with eating, swallowing, or drinking

3. A. 1. Wear disposable gloves while giving him mouth care because of risk of contact with blood from bleeding gums.
   2. Wear disposable gloves when cleaning his skin of fecal material after a bout of diarrhea because of the risk of contact with blood in the fecal material.
   3. Prepare bleach solution daily. Fresh solution is needed to maintain effectiveness. Use this solution to clean up spills of body fluids and to soak feces-stained clothing and bed linens. Bleach solution destroys the human immuno-deficiency virus.
   4. Wear disposable gloves whenever there is risk of coming into contact with bloody fluids to protect yourself from infection.
   5. Avoid splashing when disposing of the contents of the bedpan and urinal to prevent the spread of organisms. Wear a mask and goggles, if necessary.
   B. Carefully clean and dry these areas thoroughly. Record the location and size of each reddened area, and report Fernando's condition to your supervisor immediately.
   C. 1. Prepare and store foods properly.
   2. Wash fresh fruits and vegetables thoroughly.
   3. Refrigerate leftovers immediately.
   D. "No, I'm not worried about that. I've been trained to take special precautions when caring for Fernando to protect myself and to protect him from infections from others. I'm not very brave; I'm just doing my job."
   E. "Do not be afraid to touch and hug your brother. Showing affection is very important."
4. A. Notify your supervisor.
   B. Tell her to hold a pillow next to the incision and to press the area in while she coughs.
   C. Notify your supervisor.
5. A. Remove any objects that may cause the client to fall. Walk next to her to provide support and assistance as needed.
   B. Puree foods as needed, and follow the care plan for thickening foods, if necessary. Remind the client about swallowing as taught by speech-language therapist.
   C. Try to anticipate her needs, and ask questions that can be answered with a "yes" or a "no" instead of a complicated answer. Use pictures, if available.
   D. Be patient with her. Point out how well she is doing and how much she has improved.
6. Notify your supervisor immediately.

True or False

1. T
2. T
3. T
4. T
5. F Cancer treatments often cause many side effects, including the loss of hair, sores in the mouth, and bleeding gums.
6. F Parkinson's disease is a chronic illness that affects people during late middle age and older adulthood.
7. T
8. T
9. F Reasoning will not help a client with Alzheimer's disease to understand what is happening; in fact, it may confuse and agitate the client.
10. T
11. T
12. T
13. T
14. F Standard (universal) precautions are used with all clients.
15. T
16. T
17. F Clients may shower with a cast (according to the care plan), provided that the cast is wrapped in plastic and protected from water. Never soak a cast or allow a cast to become soaked.
18. F Immediately report these symptoms to your supervisor; they indicate a problem with the nerve and blood supply to the casted part.
19. T
20. T
21. F Sterile dressings are changed by the nurse.
22. F "Phantom limb pain" is real pain; it is not imagined.
23. T
24. F Too much food is overwhelming. Offer small, frequent feedings.
25. T

CHAPTER 23 CARING FOR THE CLIENT AT THE END OF LIFE

Completion

1. Clients' emotional responses to dying are (any of the following) <u>denial</u>, <u>anger</u>, <u>sadness</u>, <u>fear</u>, <u>guilt</u>, and <u>acceptance</u>.

2. A final illness from which a client is not expected to recover is called a *terminal* illness or an *end-stage disease*.

3. A living will and durable power of attorney are examples of advance directives.

4. A program that cares for the dying client and his or her caregivers is *hospice*.

5. Two signs of approaching death are slowed circulation and cold hands and feet. *(Other acceptable answers include unconsciousness, difficulty breathing, and any other symptoms listed in the text.)*

6. The last sense to leave the body is hearing.

7. Care that is provided after death is called *postmortem* care.

Situations

1. Ask Mr. Toomey why he is asking you about his death. Listen to what he says. If he doesn't understand what is happening, speak with your supervisor.

2. Discuss the situation with your supervisor to determine if your client is depressed about dying and if she is withdrawing in preparation for death. If so, your supervisor will explain the situation to the client's caregivers.

3. Even though the hope for a "miracle cure" may seem totally unrealistic, members of the health care team share that hope with clients and caregivers. If denial is present, recognize that both the client and his caregivers need that denial to cope with the emotional stresses associated with the illness.

4. Recognize Josephine's anger by saying, "Josephine, you seem to be very angry today." Then ask her to tell you about her feelings by saying, "Can you tell me how you're feeling?"

5. It's OK to be sad when your client dies. Call your agency, and speak to your supervisor about these feelings. It helps to talk about your emotions.

6. Notify your supervisor to make sure that the agency knows about these religious practices. Follow agency policy regarding the pronouncement of death. Respect the caregiver's religious practices.

7. Inform the family members that hearing is the last sense to leave the body of a dying person and that they still have time to say goodbye.

CHAPTER 24 EMERGENCIES

Completion

1. The emergency telephone number to call in my area is *(answers will vary)*.

2. Four questions that the dispatcher may ask when you report an emergency are the location of the emergency, your name and telephone number, what happened, and the condition of the victim.

3. The "Four Cs of Emergency Care" are **caution**: do not put yourself in danger, **check**: your local emergency number, **call**: your local emergency number, and **care**: for the victim until help arrives.

4. First aid situations that increase the home care aide's risk for infection are a bleeding victim, a wound that is weeping fluid, and a wound that was caused by an animal bite.

5. The four signs of a medical emergency that require immediate action are unconsciousness, no breathing, no pulse, and severe bleeding.

Situations (A)

1. A. Use a barrier to protect yourself from blood (e.g., plastic bag, plastic wrap, disposable gloves).
   B. Apply a sterile or clean dressing over the wound.
   C. Apply direct pressure over the wound.
   D. Apply a bandage snugly over the dressing to keep it in place.

2. A. Assist the victim into a position with the head lower than the legs. If injury to the back, head, or neck is suspected, keep the victim flat.
   B. Loosen any tight clothing to make breathing easier.
   C. Maintain body temperature (e.g., cover with a sweater or blanket).
   D. Reassure the victim that help is coming.

3. A. Run cool tap water over the burned area to cool the skin and to slow the burning process.
   B. Cover the burn with a dry, sterile dressing or dry, clean cloth to prevent infection.
   C. Apply loose bandage to keep the dressing in place.
   D. Do not break the blisters.

4. A. Help her to lie on the floor.
   B. Remove any furniture or other objects that the client might strike against while experiencing uncontrolled body movements.
   C. Protect her from injury.
   D. Do not restrict her movements or place anything in her mouth.

5. A. Stand behind victim, and wrap your arms around the victim's waist.
   B. Make a fist with one hand, and place the thumb side against the middle of the victim's abdomen, just above the navel and below the rib cage.
   C. Grab your fist with your other hand, and give quick, inward, and upward thrusts into the abdomen.
   D. Repeat the thrusts until the object is forced out.

6. A. Do not move the client, and ask her not to move.
   B. Maintain the client's body temperature.
   C. Remain with the client.
   D. Reassure and comfort the client.

7. A. Have him sit down immediately.
   B. Loosen any tight clothing.
   C. Reassure him that help is on the way.
   D. Help him to remain calm.

Situations (B)

1. Stop her, place her on the ground, and then roll her to smother the flames.
2. A. Adhesive tape
   B. Gauze pads
   C. Scissors
   D. Adhesive bandages
   E. Hand cleaner
   F. Disposable gloves
3. A. Take the container of toilet bowl cleaner from Louisa.
   B. Take her out of the bathroom.
   Call 9-1-1. Report the name of the toilet bowl cleaner and the time at which you found Louisa drinking the fluid.
4. A. Your client's name
   B. The type of emergency
   C. Where and when the emergency happened
   D. What first aid was given and who was called

CHAPTER 25 GETTING A JOB AND KEEPING IT

Want Ad

1. A. Experience
   B. Preferred
   C. Certification
   D. Required
   E. Excellent
   F. Reimbursement
2. A. You are reimbursed for travel while on the job.
   B. Work can occur Monday through Friday and on the weekends, too.
   C. You will be living in the client's home while providing care.
   D. Benefits include such things as medical, dental, and life insurance; paid vacation and sick days; and so on.
3. A. You would have a paper and pen handy to take notes.
   B. You would prepare a list of any general questions that you may have.

The Job Interview

1. Your appointment to be interviewed by the personnel manager of the ABC Home Care Agency is tomorrow at 1:30 PM. You should arrive at the agency no later than 1:20 PM.
2. Complete the sample application form (Workbook Figure 25-1, pp. 111–112; answers will vary).
3. Ask her to explain the travel requirements and uniforms.
4. A. 1. Give care according to the care plan.
      2. Perform the duties correctly.
   B. 1. Use the correct forms.
      2. Record client care and billable time.
   C. 1. Practice safety awareness at all times.
      2. Use standard (universal) precautions when needed.
   D. 1. Accept constructive criticism given by the supervisor.
      2. Follow suggestions for improving job performance.
5. A. 1. Provide necessary equipment and supplies to protect me from possible infection.
      2. Remove me from situations in a home where there is danger present.
   B. 1. Provide payment according to an agreed-upon rate and pay scale.
      2. Provide the correct amount of money for the time worked.
   C. 1. Regularly supervise me on the job.
      2. Respond promptly when I contact the agency to report any abnormal or unusual conditions affecting my client.
   D. 1. Inform me of the results of the evaluations.
      2. If my evaluation is not satisfactory, inform me about what will happen if my performance does not improve.
6. A. No
   B. Yes
   C. No
   D. No
   E. Yes
   F. No
   G. Yes
   H. Yes
   I. No

Crossword Puzzle

	1 J	O	B	P	L	A	C	E	M	E	N	T	C	O	U	N	S	2 E	L	O	R		3 E			
	O																	M					V			
	4 B	E	N	E	F	I	T	5 S										P					A			
	A							A										L					L			
	P							L										O					U			
	P							A										Y					A			
	L							R		6 E	M	P	L	O	Y	E	E	R	I	G	H	T	S			
	I							Y										R					I			
	C												7 M		R						O			
	A				8 C	E	R	T	I	F	I	C	A	T	I	O	N				N			
	T		9 N									N		G									
	10 I	N	T	E	R	V	I	E	W				D		H								
	O		T									A		T								
	N		W									T		S								
			O									O										
			R									R										
			K				11 E	M	P	L	O	Y	M	E	N	T	A	G	E	N	C	Y
			I																			
		12 C	O	N	T	I	N	U	I	N	G	E	D	U	C	A	T	I	O	N		
			G																			

Skills Competency Checklists

PROCEDURE 10-1. FEEDING THE CLIENT

Name: _____

	S	UN
1. Explained procedure to client.	___	___
2. Washed hands.	___	___
3. Obtained necessary materials.	___	___
4. Prepared client for mealtime:	___	___
a. Offered to assist with toileting.	___	___
b. Offered to assist client to wash hands.	___	___
c. Positioned client to sit up in bed/chair.	___	___
d. Placed table or bed tray over client's lap.	___	___
5. Draped napkin across client's chest and under chin.	___	___
6. Served food on tray, if needed.	___	___
7. Sat near client.	___	___
8. Explained what is being served.	___	___
9. Cut food, buttered bread, and prepared liquids, as needed.	___	___
10. Asked client what he/she would like to eat first.	___	___
11. Encouraged self-feeding, if appropriate.	___	___
12. Fed client one bite (i.e., one half spoonful) at a time. Allowed time for client to chew and swallow.	___	___
13. Alternated solids and liquids; used a straw, if needed.	___	___
14. Talked with client and offered praise for eating.	___	___
15. Wiped client's mouth and removed tray (if used) when client finished.	___	___
16. Washed client's face and hands. Removed napkin or bib.	___	___
17. Offered oral hygiene.	___	___
18. Made sure client was safe and comfortable.	___	___
19. Recorded in care record percent of food consumed.	___	___
20. Washed hands.	___	___
21. Washed dishes and utensils used for meal.	___	___
22. Cleaned and straightened kitchen.	___	___

Comments:

Evaluator's Signature: _____

Date: _____

PROCEDURE 11-1. HANDWASHING

Name: _____

	S	UN
1. Collected all materials at the sink.	____	____
2. Removed watch (or pushed up forearm 4 to 5 inches) and rings.	____	____
3. Stood back from sink to keep clothing from becoming wet.	____	____
4. Turned on faucet and adjusted water to comfortable temperature.	____	____
5. Wet hands and wrists completely. Kept fingers and hands below elbows.	____	____
6. Applied soap to hands.	____	____
7. Lathered hands well by rubbing palms together. Spread lather over hands and wrists, under nails, and between fingers.	____	____
8. Used rotating and rubbing motion for 30 seconds.	____	____
a. Vigorously rubbed one hand against the other and around wrist. Repeated with the other hand and wrist.	____	____
b. Washed between fingers by interlacing them.	____	____
c. Rubbed fingernails against the palms of hands.	____	____
9. Washed at least 2 inches above the wrist.	____	____
10. Rinsed well, one hand at a time. Rinsed from 2 inches above the wrist and kept hands and fingers below the elbows.	____	____
11. Dried hands and wrists with paper towels.	____	____
12. Dropped the used paper towels into wastebasket.	____	____
13. Turned off faucets using another dry paper towel.	____	____
14. Discarded towel.	____	____
15. Applied hand lotion, if desired.	____	____

Comments:

Evaluator's Signature: _____

Date: _____

PROCEDURE 11-2. APPLYING GLOVES AND REMOVING CONTAMINATED GLOVES

Name: _____

Applying Gloves	S	UN
1. Washed hands.	___	___
2. Dried hands thoroughly.	___	___
3. Inspected gloves for tears or perforations.	___	___
4. Put gloves on when ready to begin client care.	___	___

Removing Contaminated Gloves (With Both Hands Still Gloved)	S	UN
1. Used right hand to grasp glove on left hand. Grasped outer surface of glove just below the wrist cuff.	___	___
2. Pulled left glove downward until it was off and turned inside out.	___	___
3. Continued to hold left glove in right hand. Gathered up glove in right hand.	___	___
4. Inserted two fingers of left hand inside cuff of right glove. Did not touch outside of glove with bare hand.	___	___
5. Pulled right glove down, inside out, and completely over left glove.	___	___
6. Deposited both gloves in proper container.	___	___
7. Washed hands.	___	___

Comments:

Evaluator's Signature: _____

Date: _____

PROCEDURE 11-3. DISINFECTING USING WET HEAT

Name: _____

	S	UN
1. Washed hands.	___	___
2. Obtained items and placed them in pot so that all surfaces were in contact with water.	___	___
3. Covered items with water. Provided some space at top of pot for steam to escape.	___	___
4. Placed lid on top of pot.	___	___
5. Placed covered pot on stove or other source of heat. Checked to see that bottom of pot was in full contact with heat source.	___	___
6. Turned pot handle(s) to the side(s).	___	___
7. Turned on heat and brought water to a boil.	___	___
8. Boiled for 20 minutes without lifting pot lid.	___	___
9. Turned off heat.	___	___
10. Allowed water and contents to cool.	___	___
11. Removed cover with potholder.	___	___
12. Removed disinfected items. Placed on clean towel to air dry. Stored properly.	___	___
13. Washed, dried, and returned disinfecting supplies to appropriate location.	___	___
14. Washed hands.	___	___

Comments:

Evaluator's Signature: _____

Date: _____

PROCEDURE 11-4. DISINFECTING USING DRY HEAT

Name: _____

	S	UN
1. Washed hands.	___	___
2. Obtained cloth-wrapped dressings and placed them in flat pan.	___	___
3. Placed flat pan in oven.	___	___
4. Turned on oven to 350° F (180° C).	___	___
5. Allowed items to bake for 1 hour without opening oven.	___	___
6. Turned off oven and allowed items to cool.	___	___
7. Removed flat pan using pot holder.	___	___
8. Unwrapped cloth carefully without touching dressings.	___	___
9. Returned items to appropriate location.	___	___
10. Washed hands.	___	___

Comments:

Evaluator's Signature: _____

Date: _____

PROCEDURE 11-5. MAKING BLEACH SOLUTION

Name: _____

	S	UN
1. Washed hands.	____	____
2. Obtained materials needed.	____	____
3. Put on rubber utility gloves.	____	____
4. Measured 5 cups (1200 mL) of water; poured into container.	____	____
5. Measured 1/2 cup (120 mL) of household bleach; added to container.	____	____
6. Placed cap on container and shook to mix solution.	____	____
7. Prepared label, "Bleach Solution 1:10," added date and time, and applied to container.	____	____
8. Stored in closed cabinet, out of reach of children, and away from foods. Returned materials to appropriate location.	____	____
9. Removed and rinsed gloves. Hung them up to dry.	____	____
10. Washed hands.	____	____

Comments:

Evaluator's Signature: _____

Date: _____

PROCEDURE 11-6. MAKING VINEGAR SOLUTION

Name: _____

	S	UN
1. Washed hands.	___	___
2. Obtained materials needed.	___	___
3. Measured 3 cups (720 mL) of water, and poured into container.	___	___
4. Measured 1 cup (240 mL) of white vinegar, and added to container.	___	___
5. Placed cap on container and shook to mix solution.	___	___
6. Prepared label, "Vinegar Solution 1:3," dated, and applied to container.	___	___
7. Stored in closed cabinet, out of reach of children, and away from food. Returned materials to appropriate location.	___	___
8. Washed hands.	___	___

Comments:

Evaluator's Signature: _____

Date: _____

PROCEDURE 11-7. DISINFECTING WITH HOUSEHOLD SOLUTIONS

Name: _____

	S	UN
1. Washed hands.	___	___
2. Obtained materials needed.	___	___
3. Put on rubber utility gloves.	___	___
4. Washed items with detergent.	___	___
5. Rinsed items with warm water.	___	___
6. Poured solution into plastic pan.	___	___
7. Submerged washed items in solution for 10 minutes.	___	___
8. Removed items.	___	___
9. Rinsed well with hot water.	___	___
10. Laid items on paper towel to dry or hung on towel rack or shower rail to dry.	___	___
11. Cleaned area and returned materials to appropriate location.	___	___
12. Removed and rinsed gloves. Hung up to dry.	___	___
13. Washed hands.	___	___

Comments:

Evaluator's Signature: _____

Date: _____

PROCEDURE 11-8. APPLYING A MASK AND REMOVING A CONTAMINATED MASK

Name: _____

Applying a Mask	**S**	**UN**
1. Washed hands.	____	____
2. Picked up mask by top strings (or upper elastic band).	____	____
3. Positioned mask over nose and mouth, with top strings over ears. Tied strings behind head (or positioned elastic band over ears and high up on head).	____	____
4. Tied lower strings (or positioned lower elastic band low on back of head, under ears).	____	____

Removing a Contaminated Mask	**S**	**UN**
1. Washed hands.	____	____
2. Untied lower strings of mask (or pulled lower elastic band up to top of head).	____	____
3. Untied upper strings and removed mask while still holding strings (or lifted both elastic bands over head and removed mask).	____	____
4. Discarded mask in proper container.	____	____
5. Washed hands.	____	____

Comments:

Evaluator's Signature: _____

Date: _____

PROCEDURE 11-9. APPLYING A GOWN AND REMOVING A CONTAMINATED GOWN

Name: _____

Applying a Gown	**S**	**UN**
1. Washed hands.	____	____
2. Inserted arms into sleeves of gown with opening in the back.	____	____
3. Tied neck strings (or closed Velcro strips).	____	____
4. Closed back opening by overlapping one side of gown over the other.	____	____
5. Tied gown at waist (or closed Velcro strips).	____	____

Removing a Contaminated Gown	**S**	**UN**
1. Untied waist strings.	____	____
2. Untied neck strings.	____	____
3. Pulled gown down from shoulders with neck ties.	____	____
4. Leaned forward, turned gown inside out while removing it. Did not touch outside of gown.	____	____
5. Kept one hand inside sleeve of the gown and used it to pull off other sleeve. Did the same on the other side.	____	____
6. Rolled up the gown into a ball. Kept contaminated area inside.	____	____
7. Discarded gown into proper container.	____	____
8. Washed hands.	____	____

Comments:

Evaluator's Signature: _____

Date: _____

PROCEDURE 11-10. DOUBLE BAGGING

Name: _____

	S	UN
1. Obtained materials needed.	___	___
2. Had helper positioned outside of client's door with a "clean" bag. If alone, placed clean opened bag in doorway.	___	___
3. Washed hands.	___	___
4. Applied gown and gloves.	___	___
5. Entered room, took in "dirty" bag.	___	___
6. Placed contaminated materials in "dirty" bag.	___	___
7. Asked person with "clean" bag to open it for insertion of second ("dirty") bag. Helper sealed "clean" bag. If alone, placed "dirty" bag in "clean" bag without sealing it until hands are clean.	___	___
8. Removed gloves and gown. Discarded in proper container.	___	___
9. Washed hands. If alone, sealed "clean" bag containing "dirty" bag.	___	___
10. Disposed of double-bagged material properly.	___	___

Comments:

Evaluator's Signature: _____

Date: _____

PROCEDURE 12-1. RAISING CLIENT'S HEAD AND SHOULDERS

Name: _____

	S	UN
1. Explained procedure to client.	____	____
2. Washed hands.	____	____
3. Provided privacy.	____	____
4. Raised bed to convenient working height.*	____	____
5. Locked wheels on bed, or pushed bed against wall if there are no brakes.	____	____
6. Lowered rail on side of bed where aide is working.*	____	____
7. Lowered head of bed, removed pillows. Folded back top sheet.	____	____
8. Stood facing bed, with feet about 12 inches apart.	____	____
9. Asked client to place near arm under aide's near arm and shoulder. (Client's hand should reach aide's shoulder.)	____	____
10. Placed aide's near arm under client's arm and shoulder. (Aide's hand should reach client's shoulder.)	____	____
11. Slipped farthest arm under client's neck and shoulders.	____	____
12. On count of "3," aide shifted weight from foot nearest head of bed to other foot. At the same time, client was rocked to a semi-sitting position.	____	____
13. Supported client with arm locked under client's shoulder; pillows removed or readjusted using other arm.	____	____
14. Assisted client to lie back on bed using locked arms and supporting neck and shoulders as before.	____	____
15. Made sure client was safe and comfortable. Replaced top sheet.	____	____
16. Placed bed in lowest position. (Raised side rail, if indicated.)*	____	____
17. Washed hands.	____	____

Comments:

Evaluator's Signature: _____

Date: _____

---

*Will not apply if hospital bed is not used.

PROCEDURE 12-2. MOVING CLIENT TO THE SIDE OF THE BED

Name: _____

	S	UN
1. Explained procedure to client.	___	___
2. Washed hands.	___	___
3. Provided privacy.	___	___
4. Raised bed to convenient working height.*	___	___
5. Locked wheels on bed, or pushed bed against wall if there are no brakes.	___	___
6. Lowered rail on side of bed where aide is working.*	___	___
7. Folded back top sheet.	___	___
8. Stood facing bed with feet about 12 inches apart, one foot in front of the other. Shifted weight from front to rear foot as each move was performed.	___	___
9. Slipped one arm under client and reached across to the opposite shoulder. Placed other arm under middle of client's back.	___	___
10. On count of "3," aide rocked back and shifted upper segment of client's body to edge of bed.	___	___
11. Placed arms under client's waist and buttocks. Moved to edge of bed in same manner as previously described.	___	___
12. Placed arms under client's thighs and lower legs. Moved to edge of bed in same manner.	___	___
13. Made sure client is in good body alignment. Replaced top sheet.	___	___
14. Placed bed in lowest position. (Raised side rail, if indicated.)*	___	___
15. Washed hands.	___	___

Comments:

Evaluator's Signature: _____

Date: _____

---

*Will not apply if hospital bed is not used.

PROCEDURE 12-3. MOVING CLIENT UP IN BED WHEN CLIENT CAN HELP

Name: _____

	S	**UN**
1. Explained procedure to client.	____	____
2. Washed hands.	____	____
3. Provided privacy.	____	____
4. Raised bed to convenient working height.*	____	____
5. Locked wheels on bed, or pushed bed against wall if there are no brakes.	____	____
6. Lowered rail on side of bed where aide is working.*	____	____
7. Folded back top sheet. Lowered client's head; removed pillows.	____	____
8. Propped one pillow against headboard to protect client's head.	____	____
9. Stood facing head of bed, knees bent and feet about 12 inches apart.	____	____
10. Slipped one arm under client's shoulders, the other arm under client's thighs.	____	____
11. Instructed client to bend his or her knees and to firmly place feet against mattress. Gave signal to client to push with hands and feet to assist with move up in bed.	____	____
12. Helped client move toward head of bed by shifting body weight from back leg to front leg.	____	____
13. Used several small, upward moves rather than one large move to reach head of bed.	____	____
14. Made sure client is in good body alignment. Replaced top sheet and pillows.	____	____
15. Placed bed in lowest position. (Raised side rail, if indicated.)*	____	____
16. Washed hands.	____	____

Comments:

Evaluator's Signature: _____

Date: _____

---

*Will not apply if hospital bed is not used.

PROCEDURE 12-4. MOVING CLIENT UP IN BED WHEN CLIENT CANNOT HELP

Name: _____

	S	UN
1. Explained procedure to client.	___	___
2. Washed hands.	___	___
3. Provided privacy.	___	___
4. Raised bed to convenient working height.*	___	___
5. Locked wheels on bed, or pushed bed against wall if there are no brakes.	___	___
6. Lowered rail on side of bed where aide is working.*	___	___
7. Folded back top sheet. Lowered client's head; removed pillows.	___	___
8. Propped one pillow against headboard to protect client's head.	___	___
9. Made sure turning sheet was in position under client's body.	___	___
10. One person:		
a. Kept side rails up.*	___	___
b. Stood at head of bed with feet about 12 inches apart, one foot in front of the other, and faced the bed.	___	___
c. Rolled top of turning sheet toward client's head.	___	___
d. Firmly grasped top of turning sheet with both hands.	___	___
e. Used good body mechanics: bent knees and hips, kept back straight.	___	___
f. On count of "3," shifted weight from front leg to rear leg, pulled turning sheet and client up toward head of bed.	___	___
11. Two persons:		
a. Lowered both side rails.*	___	___
b. Aide took place at one side of bed with feet about 12 inches apart, one foot in front of the other, and faced head of bed. (Other person or aide did same.)	___	___
c. Sides of turning sheet were rolled close to client's body.	___	___
d. Turning sheet edges were firmly grasped with both hands.	___	___
e. Used good body mechanics: bent knees and hips, kept back straight.	___	___
f. On count of "3," aide and helper shifted body weight from rear leg to front leg, lifted turning sheet, and moved client toward head of bed.	___	___
12. Checked lower sheets for wrinkles; smoothed, if necessary.	___	UN
13. Made sure client was in good body alignment. Replaced top sheet and pillows.	___	___
14. Placed bed in lowest position. (Raised side rail, if indicated.)*	___	___
15. Washed hands.	___	___

Comments:

Evaluator's Signature: _____

Date: _____

---

*Will not apply if hospital bed is not used.

PROCEDURE 12-5. POSITIONING CLIENT IN THE SUPINE (BACK-LYING) POSITION

Name: _____

	S	UN
1. Explained procedure to client.	___	___
2. Washed hands.	___	___
3. Provided privacy.	___	___
4. Raised bed to convenient working height.*	___	___
5. Locked wheels on bed, or pushed bed against wall if there are no brakes.	___	___
6. Lowered rail on side of bed where aide is working.*	___	___
7. Folded back top sheet. Positioned client on back.	___	___
8. Adjusted pillows properly:	___	___
a. Small pillow under head and shoulders.	___	___
b. Supported arms and hands with pillows.	___	___
c. Small pillow or folded towel placed under small of back (if supervisor so instructed).	___	___
9. Positioned other devices, such as footboard, trochanter rolls, bed cradle, as indicated in care plan.	___	___
10. Made sure client is in proper body alignment. Replaced top sheet.	___	___
11. Placed bed in lowest position. (Raised side rail, if indicated.)*	___	___
12. Washed hands.	___	___
13. Recorded what was done.	___	___

Comments:

Evaluator's Signature: _____

Date: _____

_____
*Will not apply if hospital bed is not used.

PROCEDURE 12-6. POSITIONING CLIENT IN THE FOWLER'S (SEMI-SITTING) POSITION

Name: _____

	S	UN
1. Explained procedure to client.	___	___
2. Washed hands.	___	___
3. Provided privacy.	___	___
4. Raised bed to convenient working height.*	___	___
5. Locked wheels on bed, or pushed bed against wall if there are no brakes.	___	___
6. Lowered rail on side of bed where aide is working.*	___	___
7. Folded back top sheet. Positioned client on back.	___	___
8. Raised head of bed to 45-degree angle. If bed was not adjustable, used other devices to position client.	___	___
9. Adjusted pillows properly:	___	___
a. Small pillow under head and shoulders.	___	___
b. Supported arms and hands with pillows.	___	___
10. Positioned other devices, such as footboard, trochanter rolls, bed cradle, as indicated in care plan.	___	___
11. Made sure client is in proper body alignment. Replaced top sheet.	___	___
12. Placed bed in lowest position. (Raised side rail, if indicated.)*	___	___
13. Washed hands.	___	___
14. Recorded what was done.	___	___

Comments:

Evaluator's Signature: _____

Date: _____

---

*Will not apply if hospital bed is not used.

PROCEDURE 12-7. POSITIONING CLIENT IN THE LATERAL (SIDE-LYING) POSITION

Name: _____

	S	UN
1. Explained procedure to client.	___	___
2. Washed hands.	___	___
3. Provided privacy.	___	___
4. Raised bed to convenient working height.*	___	___
5. Locked wheels on bed, or pushed bed against wall if there are no brakes.	___	___
6. Lowered rail on side of bed where aide is working.*	___	___
7. Lowered client's head and removed pillows. Folded back top sheet.	___	___
8. Asked client to move to side of bed nearest aide. Assisted client, as needed.	___	___
9. Raised side rail.*	___	___
10. Went to other side of bed and lowered side rail.*	___	___
11. Placed one hand around client's farthest shoulder and other hand around client's farthest hip. Rolled client toward aide and turned client on side facing toward center of bed. Bent client's upper leg and both arms.	___	___
12. Adjusted pillows properly:	___	___
a. Small pillow under head and neck.	___	___
b. Supported upper arm and leg on pillows.	___	___
c. Folded towel placed along back to maintain side-lying position (optional).	___	___
13. Positioned other devices as indicated in care plan.	___	___
14. Made sure client is in good body alignment. Replaced top sheet.	___	___
15. Placed bed in lowest position. (Raised side rail, if indicated.)*	___	___
16. Washed hands.	___	___
17. Recorded what was done.	___	___

Comments:

Evaluator's Signature: _____

Date: _____

*Will not apply if hospital bed is not used.

PROCEDURE 12-8. POSITIONING CLIENT IN THE SIMS' POSITION

Name: _____

	S	UN
1. Explained procedure to client.	___	___
2. Washed hands.	___	___
3. Provided privacy.	___	___
4. Raised bed to convenient working height.*	___	___
5. Locked wheels on bed, or pushed bed against wall if there are no brakes.	___	___
6. Lowered rail on side of bed where aide is working.*	___	___
7. Lowered client's head; removed pillows. Folded back top sheet.	___	___
8. Asked client to move to side of bed nearest aide. Assisted client as needed.	___	___
9. Raised side rail.*	___	___
10. Went to other side of bed and lowered side rail.*	___	___
11. Placed one hand around client's farthest shoulder and other hand around client's farthest hip. Rolled client toward aide and turned client on side facing toward center of bed. Positioned upper leg so it did not rest on lower leg. (Lower arm should be behind client.)	___	___
12. Adjusted pillows properly:	___	___
a. Small pillow under head and neck.	___	___
b. Supported upper arm and leg on pillows.	___	___
13. Positioned other devices as indicated in care plan.	___	___
14. Made sure client is in good body alignment. Replaced top sheet.	___	___
15. Placed bed in lowest position. (Raised side rail, if indicated.)*	___	___
16. Washed hands.	___	___
17. Recorded what was done. Reported any unusual conditions to supervisor.	___	___

Comments:

Evaluator's Signature: _____

Date: _____

---

*Will not apply if hospital bed is not used.

PROCEDURE 12-9. POSITIONING CLIENT IN THE PRONE (ABDOMINAL) POSITION

Name: _____

	S	UN
1. Explained procedure to client.	____	____
2. Washed hands.	____	____
3. Provided privacy.	____	____
4. Raised bed to convenient working height.*	____	____
5. Locked wheels on bed, or pushed bed against wall if there are no brakes.	____	____
6. Lowered rail on side of bed where aide is working.*	____	____
7. Lowered client's head; removed pillows. Folded back top sheet.	____	____
8. Asked client to move to side of bed nearest aide. Assisted client, as needed.	____	____
9. Raised side rail.*	____	____
10. Went to other side of bed and lowered side rail.*	____	____
11. Placed one hand around client's farthest shoulder and other hand around client's farthest hip. Rolled client toward aide and turned client on side and then onto abdomen. Turned client's head to side with arms flexed on each side of client's head.	____	____
12. Adjusted pillows properly:	____	____
a. Small pillow under head and neck.	____	____
b. Optional small pillow under abdomen.	____	____
c. Pillow placed under lower legs to relieve pressure on toes. Client may be positioned so that toes hang over mattress.	____	____
13. Made sure client is in good body alignment. Replaced top sheet.	____	____
14. Placed bed in lowest position. (Raised side rail, if indicated.)*	____	____
15. Washed hands.	____	____
16. Recorded what was done. Reported any unusual conditions to supervisor.	____	____

Comments:

Evaluator's Signature: _____

Date: _____

_____
*Will not apply if hospital bed is not used.

PROCEDURE 12-10. ASSISTING CLIENT TO SIT ON THE SIDE OF THE BED

Name: _____

	S	UN
1. Explained procedure to client.	___	___
2. Washed hands.	___	___
3. Obtained necessary materials.	___	___
4. Provided privacy.	___	___
5. Raised bed to convenient working height.*	___	___
6. Locked wheels on bed, or pushed bed against wall if there are no brakes.	___	___
7. Lowered rail on side of bed where aide is working.*	___	___
8. Folded back top bedding.	___	___
9. Stood as close to side of bed as possible (legs touching side of bed) and was level with client.	___	___
10. Positioned feet apart, with one foot staggered. Bent hips and knees.	___	___
11. Asked client to move to side of bed nearest aide. Assisted client, as needed.	___	___
12. Put up side rail and raised head of bed.*	___	___
13. Placed client in Fowler's position, without pillows.	___	___
14. Lowered bed and put side rail down.*	___	___
15. Placed one arm around client's shoulder area and other arm under client's knees.	___	___
16. On count of "3," shifted weight to rear leg and slowly swung client's legs over edge of bed while pulling shoulders to sitting position.	___	___
17. Placed bed in lowest position so client's feet touched floor.*	___	___
18. Remained facing client with both hands supporting shoulders until client was stable.	___	___
19. Assisted client to put on robe and footwear. Applied transfer or gait belt, if needed, for transfer.	___	___
20. Placed back of chair next to bed, facing client. Had client hold back of chair to keep balance, if needed.	___	___
21. Remained with client.	___	___
22. Reversed procedure to return client to Fowler's position.	___	___
23. Washed hands.	___	___
24. Recorded client's reaction to procedure, amount of time spent sitting on side of bed, and any other observations.	___	___

Comments:

Evaluator's Signature: _____

Date: _____

*Will not apply if hospital bed is not used.

PROCEDURE 12-11. TRANSFERRING CLIENT FROM BED TO CHAIR/WHEELCHAIR: STANDING TRANSFER

Name: _____

	S	UN
1. Explained procedure to client.	___	___
2. Washed hands.	___	___
3. Obtained necessary materials.	___	___
4. Provided privacy.	___	___
5. Placed chair parallel to bed on client's strong side.	___	___
6. If wheelchair was used, locked brakes and moved footrests out of the way.	___	___
7. Lowered bed, locked wheels, and lowered side rail.*	___	___
8. Assisted client, as needed, to sit on side of bed and to put on robe and footwear.	___	___
9. Stood directly in front of client, with feet slightly apart. Bent hips and knees to be level with client.	___	___
10. Placed arms under client's arms and around client's back, locking fingers together or clasping one hand over the other wrist. Asked client to hug aide's back (not aide's neck).	___	___
11. Locked knees against client's knees to provide additional support and to prevent the knees from buckling.	___	___
12. Bent knees and asked client to rock with aide while counting 1-2-3. Stood on the count of "3."	___	___
13. Counted to 10 before continuing to allow the client time to adjust to standing position.	___	___
14. Walked with client to chair (took small steps) and guided client's back to chair. Continued until chair's sitting surface touched back of client's legs.	___	___
15. Had client reach back and grasp the farthest arm of the chair, then the nearest arm.	___	___
16. Bent hips and knees while guiding client into chair.	___	___
17. Made sure client was safe and comfortable.	___	___
a. If helping client into wheelchair, replaced footrests, and had client put feet on them.	___	___
b. Placed necessary items within client's reach.	___	___
18. Washed hands.	___	___
19. Recorded client's reaction to procedure, amount of time spent sitting in chair, and any other observations.	___	___

Comments:

Evaluator's Signature: _____

Date: _____

---

*Will not apply if hospital bed is not used.

PROCEDURE 12-12. TRANSFERRING CLIENT FROM BED TO CHAIR/WHEELCHAIR: STANDING TRANSFER USING TRANSFER BELT

Name: _____

	S	UN
1. Explained procedure to client.	___	___
2. Washed hands.	___	___
3. Obtained materials needed.	___	___
4. Provided privacy.	___	___
5. Applied transfer belt.	___	___
6. Placed chair parallel to bed and on client's strong side. If wheelchair was used, locked brakes and moved footrests out of the way. If bed had wheels, locked them.	___	___
7. Stood directly in front of client.	___	___
8. Made sure client's feet were firmly on the floor.	___	___
9. Had client place fists on bed next to thighs and lean forward.	___	___
10. Grasped transfer belt firmly at each side.	___	___
11. Locked knees against client's knees to provide additional support and to prevent client's knees from buckling.	___	___
12. Asked client to push fists down on bed and stand on count of "3."	___	___
13. Pulled client to standing position while straightening knees and legs.	___	___
14. Counted to 10 before continuing.	___	___
15. Instructed client to:	___	___
a. Take small steps while turning back to chair until legs touch the chair.	___	___
b. Reach back and grasp the farthest arm of the chair, then the nearest arm.	___	___
c. Lower buttocks into chair, leaning slightly forward while sitting down.	___	___
d. Slide buttocks to back of chair and sit erect.	___	___
16. Made sure client was safe and comfortable.	___	___
a. If in wheelchair, replaced footrests and had client put feet on them.	___	___
b. Placed necessary items within client's reach.	___	___
17. Washed hands.	___	___
18. Recorded client's reaction to procedure, amount of time spent sitting in chair, and any other observations.	___	___

Comments:

Evaluator's Signature: _____

Date: _____

———————

*Will not apply if hospital bed is not used.

PROCEDURE 12-13. RETURNING CLIENT TO BED

Name: _____

	S	UN
1. Explained procedure to client.	___	___
2. Washed hands.	___	___
3. Provided privacy.	___	___
4. Prepared bed; folded down top bedding.	___	___
5. Lowered height of bed to lowest level.*	___	___
6. Placed chair parallel to bed; client moved toward strong side.	___	___
7. If wheelchair was used, locked brakes and moved footrests out of the way. Locked bed wheels (if present).	___	___
8. Directed client to:	___	___
a. Hold on to armrests.	___	___
b. Slide to edge of chair.	___	___
c. Push down on armrests, straighten legs, and stand up.	___	___
d. Take small steps while turning back to bed until back of legs touch bed.	___	___
e. Reach back and place hands on bed.	___	___
f. Lower buttocks onto bed and slide back in bed.	___	___
9. Assisted client to remove robe and shoes.	___	___
10. Made sure client was safe and comfortable.	___	___
11. Placed bed in lowest position. (Raised side rails, if indicated.)*	___	___
12. Washed hands.	___	___
13. Recorded what was done and client's reaction.	___	___

Comments:

Evaluator's Signature: _____

Date: _____

---

*Will not apply if hospital bed is not used.

PROCEDURE 12-14. APPLYING A TRANSFER (GAIT) BELT

Name: _____

	S	UN
1. Explained procedure to client.	____	____
2. Washed hands.	____	____
3. Obtained transfer (gait) belt.	____	____
4. Assisted client to sitting position on side of bed.	____	____
5. Applied belt over client's clothing and around waist.	____	____
6. Placed belt buckles off-center in the front or in the back, according to client's comfort.	____	____
7. Tightened belt, using buckles, until it was snug.	____	____
8. Checked that breasts (women) were not caught in the belt.	____	____
9. Prepared client for transfer.	____	____

Comments:

Evaluator's Signature: _____

Date: _____

PROCEDURE 12-15. USING A MECHANICAL LIFT

Name: _____

	S	UN
1. Explained procedure to client.	____	____
2. Washed hands.	____	____
3. Obtained necessary materials.	____	____
4. Provided privacy.	____	____
5. Raised bed to convenient working height and lowered side rails.*	____	____
6. Lowered head of bed to level that was comfortable for client and as low as possible.*	____	____
7. Centered sling with sheet on top, placing them underneath client by turning client from side to side.	____	____
8. Positioned sling according to manufacturer's instructions.	____	____
9. Placed chair/wheelchair at head or foot of bed, about 1 foot away from side of bed.	____	____
10. Locked wheels on bed.*	____	____
11. Raised lift and positioned it over client.	____	____
12. Rolled base of lift under bed, locating swivel bar over client.	____	____
13. Attached sling to swivel bar.	____	____
14. Raised head of bed to sitting position.*	____	____
15. Placed client's arms across his or her chest. Client did not touch swivel bar.	____	____
16. Pumped lift high enough for client and sling to be free of bed.	____	____
17. Asked helper to support client's legs and guide client as lift was moved and client moved away from bed.	____	____
18. Positioned lift so that client's back was toward chair.	____	____
19. Lowered client into chair as helper guided client into chair. Followed manufacturer's instructions for lowering lift.	____	____
20. Lowered swivel bar to unhook sling. Left sling in place.	____	____
21. Put on client's footwear; positioned feet.	____	____
22. Covered client's lap and legs with blanket, as needed.	____	____
23. Made sure client was safe and comfortable.	____	____
24. Washed hands.	____	____
25. Recorded client's reaction to procedure, amount of time spent sitting in chair, and any other observations.	____	____
26. Reversed procedure to return client to bed.	____	____

Comments:

Evaluator's Signature: _____

Date: _____

_____
*Will not apply if hospital bed is not used.

PROCEDURE 13-1. MAKING A CLOSED BED

Name: _____

	S	UN
1. Explained procedure to client.	___	___
2. Washed hands.	___	___
3. Obtained materials needed and placed them in order of use on chair near bed.	___	___
4. Placed laundry container near bed.	___	___
5. Raised bed to convenient working height, and lowered both rails.*	___	___
6. Placed bed in flat position.*	___	___
7. Removed pillow(s) and placed on chair.	___	___
8. Loosened all bed linens—at head, sides, and bottom of bed.	___	___
9. Removed each piece of bed linen separately. Folded any linens to be reused. Rolled each remaining linen into a ball and discarded in laundry container.	___	___
10. Placed clean mattress pad, folded lengthwise, in center of bed. Unfolded one half of pad and rolled to center of bed.†	___	___
11. Placed bottom sheet, folded lengthwise, in center of bed. Unfolded one half and rolled to center of bed.	___	___
• Fitted sheet: placed ends around corners, top and bottom, then tucked side of sheet under mattress.	___	___
• Flat sheet: placed bottom hem of sheet even with edge of mattress at foot of bed; tucked top of sheet under mattress at head of bed.	___	___
12. Mitered corner at head of mattress.	___	___
13. Tucked sheet under side of entire mattress. Worked from head of bed to foot of bed.	___	___
14. Placed plastic drawsheet, folded in half, in center third of bed. Unfolded and rolled to center of bed.†	___	___
15. Placed cotton drawsheet, folded in half, in center of bed, covering entire plastic drawsheet. Unfolded and rolled it to center of bed.†	___	___
16. Tucked ends of plastic drawsheet and cotton drawsheet under mattress.†	___	___
17. Placed top sheet, folded lengthwise, in center of bed, with top edge even with top of mattress. Unfolded and rolled it to center of bed.	___	___
18. Placed blanket, folded lengthwise, in center of bed, with top edge even with top of mattress. Unfolded and rolled it to center of bed.†	___	___
19. Placed bedspread, folded lengthwise, in center of bed, with about 4 inches above the top edge of the mattress. Unfolded and rolled it to center of bed.†	___	___
20. Tucked top sheet, blanket, and bedspread under foot of mattress. Mitered corner.	___	___
21. Went to other side of bed.	___	___
22. Pulled through mattress pad and straightened.†	___	___
23. Pulled through all lower linens. Straightened and tucked under mattress. Mitered corner of sheet at head of bed (or placed top and bottom corners of fitted sheet over mattress corners).	___	___

24. Pulled through top sheet, blanket, and bedspread. Smoothed out wrinkles.   ____ ____

25. Tucked top sheet, blanket, and bedspread under foot of mattress.   ____ ____

26. Mitered corner at foot of bed.   ____ ____

27. Made a cuff at top of bed and brought top sheet over blanket.   ____ ____

28. Placed clean pillowcase on pillow and placed pillow at head of bed.   ____ ____

29. Covered pillow with bedspread.   ____ ____

30. Placed bed in lowest position.*   ____ ____

31. Removed laundry container and took to washing machine or other location as requested by client or family.   ____ ____

32. Washed hands.   ____ ____

Comments:

Evaluator's Signature: _____

Date: _____

---

*Will not apply if hospital bed is not used.
†Optional.

PROCEDURE 13-2. MAKING AN OPEN BED

Name: _____

	S	UN
1. Washed hands.	____	____
2. Obtained materials needed.	____	____
3. Made a closed bed.	____	____
4. Fanfolded top linens to foot of bed.	____	____
5. Washed hands.	____	____

Comments:

Evaluator's Signature: _____

Date: _____

PROCEDURE 13-3. MAKING AN OCCUPIED BED

Name: _____

		S	UN
1.	Explained procedure to client.	___	___
2.	Washed hands.	___	___
3.	Obtained materials needed and placed them in order of use on chair near bed.	___	___
4.	Provided privacy.	___	___
5.	Placed laundry container near bed.	___	___
6.	Raised bed to convenient working height and locked wheels. Lowered rail on side of bed where aide is working.*	___	___
7.	Lowered head of bed as low as possible to level comfortable for client.*	___	___
8.	Loosened top bedding at foot of bed.	___	___
9.	Removed top bedding (bedspread, quilt) but left client covered with one blanket or top sheet.	___	___
10.	Instructed client to hold top sheet while other top linens removed.	___	___
11.	Folded any linens to be reused, such as blanket or quilt. Rolled each remaining linen into a ball and discarded in laundry container.	___	___
12.	Helped client to roll to side of bed opposite aide and grasp side rail for support.*	___	___
13.	Rolled each piece of bottom linen to center of bed and tucked along client's back.	___	___
14.	Smoothed mattress pad, if used.†	___	___
15.	Placed clean bottom sheet, folded lengthwise, in center of bed. Unfolded one half and rolled it to center of bed.	___	___
	• Fitted sheet: placed ends around corners, top and bottom; tucked side of sheet under mattress.	___	___
	• Flat sheet: placed bottom hem of sheet even with edge of mattress at foot of bed; tucked top of sheet under mattress at head of bed.	___	___
16.	Mitered corner at head of mattress.	___	___
17.	Tucked sheet under side of entire mattress. Worked from head of bed to foot of bed.	___	___
18.	Placed plastic drawsheet, folded in half, in center third of bed. Unfolded and rolled to center of bed. Tucked along client's back.†	___	___
19.	Placed cotton drawsheet, folded in half, in center of bed, covering entire plastic drawsheet. Unfolded and rolled it to center of bed. Tucked along client's back.	___	___
20.	Tucked ends of drawsheet(s) under mattress.†	___	___
21.	Helped client to roll toward aide; over linens to clean side of bed.	___	___
22.	Raised rail on side where aide was working.*	___	___
23.	Went to other side of bed.	___	___
24.	Lowered side rail.*	___	___
25.	Removed used bottom linens, rolled, and discarded in laundry container.	___	___

26. Pulled through all bottom linens. Straightened and tucked under head of mattress. Mitered corner of sheet at head of bed (Or fitted top and bottom corners of fitted sheet over mattress corners.)   ____ ____

27. Helped client to roll back to center of bed.   ____ ____

28. Placed clean top sheet entirely over client and removed top linens; discarded in laundry container or folded for reuse.   ____ ____

29. Placed blanket and bedspread over sheet.   ____ ____

30. Tucked top sheet, blanket, and bedspread under foot of mattress. Made a mitered corner.   ____ ____

31. Raised side rail.*   ____ ____

32. Went to other side of bed. Lowered side rail.*   ____ ____

33. Smoothed and straightened top sheet, blanket, and bedspread. Tucked them under foot of mattress. Provided toe room. Made a mitered corner.   ____ ____

34. Made cuff at top of bed and brought top sheet over bedspread.   ____ ____

35. Removed pillow from bed, took off case, and discarded case in laundry container.   ____ ____

36. Applied clean pillowcase; placed pillow under client's head.   ____ ____

37. Made sure client was safe and comfortable.   ____ ____

38. Placed bed in lowest position. (Raise side rail, if indicated.)*   ____ ____

39. Removed laundry container to proper location.   ____ ____

40. Washed hands.   ____ ____

Comments:

Evaluator's Signature: _____

Date: _____

---

*Will not apply if hospital bed is not used.
†Optional.

PROCEDURE 13-4. MAKING A MITERED CORNER

Name: _____

Bottom Bedding	S	UN
1. Tucked bottom sheet about 18 inches under mattress at head of bed.	____	____
2. Turned side of sheet up over mattress in a triangle shape.	____	____
3. Tucked lower edge of sheet (hanging down next to the mattress) under side of mattress.	____	____
4. Turned triangular area of sheet down over mattress.	____	____
5. Tucked sheet under mattress.	____	____

Comments:

Evaluator's Signature: _____

Date: _____

PROCEDURE 14-1. BRUSHING TEETH

Name: _____

	S	UN
1. Explained procedure to client.	____	____
2. Washed hands.	____	____
3. Obtained necessary materials.	____	____
4. Provided privacy.	____	____
5. Spread paper towel on work area. Arranged supplies on paper towel.	____	____
6. Raised bed to convenient working height. Lowered rail on side of bed.*	____	____
7. Assisted client to an upright position, or turned on side if unable to sit up.	____	____
8. Placed face towel under client's chin and over chest.	____	____
9. Put on gloves.	____	____
10. Assisted client with self-care as necessary.	____	____
11. Held toothbrush over emesis basin and poured a little water over the brush to moisten. Applied toothpaste.	____	____
12. Brushed client's teeth (if client was unable to do so).	____	____
13. Had client rinse mouth with water. Held emesis basin so client could spit into it.	____	____
14. Had client rinse with mouthwash (optional). Held emesis basin so client could spit into it.	____	____
15. Wiped client's mouth with face towel.	____	____
16. Removed face towel.	____	____
17. Removed and discarded gloves.	____	____
18. Made sure client was safe and comfortable.	____	____
19. Placed bed in lowest position. (Raised side rail, if indicated.)*	____	____
20. Cleaned equipment and stored in proper location.	____	____
21. Wiped work surface with paper towel and discarded.	____	____
22. Placed soiled face towel in laundry container to be washed.	____	____
23. Washed hands.	____	____
24. Recorded what was done. Reported any unusual conditions to supervisor.	____	____

Comments:

Evaluator's Signature: _____

Date: _____

---

*Will not apply if hospital bed is not used.

PROCEDURE 14-2. FLOSSING TEETH

Name: _____

	S	UN
1. Explained procedure to client.	____	____
2. Washed hands.	____	____
3. Obtained necessary materials.	____	____
4. Provided privacy.	____	____
5. Spread paper towel on work area. Arranged supplies on paper towel.	____	____
6. Raised bed to convenient working height. Lowered rail on side of bed.*	____	____
7. Assisted client to upright position, or turned on side if unable to sit up.	____	____
8. Placed face towel under client's chin and over chest.	____	____
9. Put on gloves.	____	____
10. Removed 18 inches (44 to 46 cm) of floss from dispenser.	____	____
11. Wrapped floss around middle finger of each hand to clean upper teeth.	____	____
12. Held floss with index fingers to clean lower teeth.	____	____
13. Inserted floss between teeth and used up-and-down, back-and-forth motions to remove material between teeth. Proceeded from tooth to tooth in the following order:	____	____
a. Upper teeth, left to right	____	____
b. Lower teeth, left to right	____	____
14. Had client rinse mouth with water. Held emesis basin so client could spit into it.	____	____
15. Wiped client's mouth with face towel.	____	____
16. Removed face towel.	____	____
17. Removed and discarded gloves.	____	____
18. Made sure client was safe and comfortable.	____	____
19. Placed bed in lowest position. (Raised side rail, if indicated.)*	____	____
20. Cleaned equipment and stored in proper location.	____	____
21. Wiped work surface with paper towel and discarded.	____	____
22. Placed soiled face towel in laundry container to be washed.	____	____
23. Washed hands.	____	____
24. Recorded what was done. Reported any unusual conditions to supervisor.	____	____

Comments:

Evaluator's Signature: _____

Date: _____

_____
*Will not apply if hospital bed is not used.

PROCEDURE 14-3. MOUTH CARE FOR THE UNCONSCIOUS CLIENT

Name: _____

	S	UN
1. Explained procedure to client.	___	___
2. Washed hands.	___	___
3. Obtained necessary materials.	___	___
4. Provided privacy.	___	___
5. Spread paper towel on work area. Arranged supplies on paper towel.	___	___
6. Raised bed to convenient working height. Lowered rail on side.*	___	___
7. Placed client in side-lying position.	___	___
8. Placed face towel and emesis basin under client's chin.	___	___
9. Put on gloves.	___	___
10. Gently opened client's mouth with padded tongue depressor.	___	___
11. Moistened foam swab and cleaned all surfaces of client's mouth: roof of mouth, tongue, gums, lips, insides of cheeks. Rinsed and re-wet swab as necessary. Cleaned teeth with swab.	___	___
12. Wiped client's mouth with face towel.	___	___
13. Removed face towel.	___	___
14. Applied lubricant to client's lips.	___	___
15. Removed and discarded gloves.	___	___
16. Made sure client was safe and comfortable.	___	___
17. Placed bed in lowest position. (Raised side rail, if indicated.)*	___	___
18. Cleaned equipment and stored in proper location.	___	___
19. Wiped work surface with paper towel and discarded.	___	___
20. Placed soiled face towel in laundry container to be washed.	___	___
21. Washed hands.	___	___
22. Recorded what was done. Reported any unusual conditions to supervisor.	___	___

Comments:

Evaluator's Signature: _____

Date: _____

---

*Will not apply if hospital bed is not used.

PROCEDURE 14-4. CARING FOR DENTURES

Name: _____

	S	UN
1. Explained procedure to client.	____	____
2. Washed hands.	____	____
3. Obtained necessary materials.	____	____
4. Provided privacy.	____	____
5. Spread paper towel on work area. Arranged supplies on paper towel (if procedure performed at bedside) or took supplies for cleaning dentures to sink.	____	____
6. Raised bed to convenient working height. Lowered side rail.*	____	____
7. Assisted client to upright position or turned on side if unable to sit up.	____	____
8. Put on gloves.	____	____
9. Asked client to remove dentures and placed in emesis basin. If dentures must be removed by aide, used gauze or a tissue as follows:	____	____
a. Upper dentures: Grasped dentures between thumb and index finger and moved up and down gently. Pulled down and removed.	____	____
b. Lower dentures: Grasped in the same manner and gently twisted sideways and up, lifting them out of the mouth.	____	____
10. Assisted client to brush dentures.	____	____
11. Cleaned dentures at sink:	____	____
a. Partially filled sink with warm water.	____	____
b. Brushed with warm water and toothpaste in an up-and-down motion. Rinsed thoroughly.	____	____
12. Returned dentures to client for replacement in the mouth or stored in denture cup.	____	____
13. Removed and discarded gloves.	____	____
14. Made sure client was safe and comfortable.	____	____
15. Placed bed in lowest position. (Raised side rail, if indicated.)*	____	____
16. Cleaned equipment and stored in proper location.	____	____
17. Wiped work surface with paper towel and discarded.	____	____
18. Washed hands.	____	____
19. Recorded what was done. Reported any unusual conditions to supervisor.	____	____

Comments:

Evaluator's Signature: _____

Date: _____

---

*Will not apply if hospital bed is not used.

PROCEDURE 14-5. GIVING A COMPLETE BED BATH

Name: _____

	S	UN
1. Explained procedure to client.	___	___
2. Washed hands.	___	___
3. Obtained necessary materials.	___	___
4. Provided privacy.	___	___
5. Raised bed to convenient working height. Locked wheels. Lowered rail on side.*	___	___
6. Offered bedpan or urinal.	___	___
7. Lowered head of bed as low as possible to level comfortable for client.*	___	___
8. Removed top bedding and covered client with bath blanket or top sheet.	___	___
9. Helped client to remove clothing, if needed.	___	___
10. Helped client to move to side of bed near aide.	___	___
11. Helped client with oral hygiene, if needed.	___	___
12. Filled wash basin two-thirds full with warm water (110° to 115° F; 43° to 46° C).	___	___
13. Placed towel under client's head and towel over client's chest.	___	___
14. Made a mitt with washcloth to be used throughout procedure.	___	___
15. Washed eye areas gently with clean water only. Started from inner corner of eye to outer corner of eye. Used opposite corners of washcloth for each eye.	___	___
16. Asked client if he or she preferred soap or cleansing cream to clean face.	___	___
17. Washed face from center outward. Used firm, gentle movements.	___	___
18. Washed ears and neck. Rinsed and dried using towel on client's chest.	___	___
19. Put a towel, lengthwise, under the arm and a towel near hand on which to place the wash basin.	___	___
20. Put client's hand in basin; allowed it to soak. Washed the arm and armpit.	___	___
21. Washed, rinsed, and dried arm, armpit, and hand. Applied deodorant under the arm, if requested. Pushed back cuticles; cleaned under nails with orangewood stick. Dried between fingers thoroughly.	___	___
22. Followed steps 19 to 21 for the other arm and hand.	___	___
23. Placed basin back on bedside table or chair.	___	___
24. Put towel over chest and abdomen. Pulled bath blanket (top sheet) to thighs. Did not expose client when washing chest and abdomen.	___	___
25. Washed, rinsed, and dried chest and abdomen. Covered chest and abdomen with bath blanket (top sheet). Removed towel.	___	___
26. Uncovered leg. Did not expose genital area. Placed towel under the leg and foot. Placed another towel near foot and put basin on towel.	___	___
27. Bent client's knee and put foot in basin; allowed it to soak. Washed and dried leg while foot was soaking.	___	___

28. Washed and dried foot. Cleaned under toenails. Dried between toes thoroughly. ____ ____

29. Repeated steps 26 to 28 for other leg and foot. ____ ____

30. Placed basin back on bedside table or chair. ____ ____

31. Turned client on side; draped bath blanket (top sheet) and exposed back and buttocks. ____ ____

32. Placed towel on bed, tucked lengthwise along neck and shoulders to buttocks. ____ ____

33. Washed, rinsed, and dried neck, shoulders, back, and buttocks. Worked from neck to buttocks. Used long strokes for washing the back. ____ ____

34. Gave back rub. ____ ____

35. Changed bath water. ____ ____

36. Turned client onto back. ____ ____

37. Placed towel under buttocks. Placed basin, soap, and towels within reach. Had client wash his or her own genital and rectal areas. Asked client to tell you when this was complete. If client was unable to wash these areas, aide completed this part of the bath wearing disposable gloves. ____ ____

38. Helped client to put on gown, pajamas, or other clothing. ____ ____

39. Combed or brushed client's hair. ____ ____

40. Made sure client was safe and comfortable. ____ ____

41. Placed bed in lowest position. (Raised side rail, if indicated.)* ____ ____

42. Emptied and cleaned wash basin. Wiped off work area with paper towels and discarded. Placed soiled towels and washcloth in laundry container to be washed. Returned other supplies to their proper place. ____ ____

43. Washed hands. ____ ____

44. Recorded what was done. Reported any unusual conditions to supervisor. ____ ____

Comments:

Evaluator's Signature: _____

Date: _____

---

*Will not apply if hospital bed is not used.

PROCEDURE 14-6. GIVING A TUB BATH

Name: _____

	S	UN
1. Explained procedure to client.	___	___
2. Washed hands.	___	___
3. Obtained necessary materials.	___	___
4. Prepared bathroom by placing skid-proof mat on bottom of tub, making sure room was warm and free of drafts, and placing straight chair in bathroom.	___	___
5. Provided privacy.	___	___
6. Helped client to undress, put on bathrobe and footwear. Placed client in wheelchair, if used. Locked brakes and put footrests in place.	___	___
7. Filled tub one-third full of warm water (110° to 115° F; 43° to 46° C).	___	___
8. Helped client to bathroom and closed door.	___	___
9. Placed client in chair facing tub. If wheelchair was used, locked brakes and placed footrests out of the way.	___	___
10. Helped client to lift one foot and then the other over the side of the tub.	___	___
11. Helped client to lower into the water; used grab bars for support.	___	___
12. Helped client to bathe, as needed.	___	___
13. Drained water from tub before getting client out of tub.	___	___
14. Helped client to dry body. Assisted client to put on bathrobe or covered with dry towel.	___	___
15. Placed straight chair or wheelchair facing tub, and placed dry towel on side of tub.	___	___
16. Helped client to sit on towel on side of tub using grab bars.	___	___
17. Helped client to stand, get out of tub and into straight chair or wheelchair, and put on footwear.	___	___
18. Helped client to room.	___	___
19. Gave a back rub.	___	___
20. Helped client to put on clean clothing and return to bed, sofa, etc. Placed in comfortable position.	___	___
21. Made sure client was safe and comfortable.	___	___
22. Returned to bathroom. Cleaned tub and straightened area.	___	___
23. Placed soiled towels and washcloth in laundry container to be washed.	___	___
24. Washed hands.	___	___
25. Recorded what was done. Reported any unusual conditions to supervisor.	___	___

Comments:

Evaluator's Signature: _____

Date: _____

PROCEDURE 14-7. GIVING A BACK RUB

Name: _____

	S	UN
1. Explained procedure to client.	____	____
2. Washed hands.	____	____
3. Obtained necessary materials.	____	____
4. Provided privacy.	____	____
5. Raised bed to convenient working height and locked wheels. Lowered rail on side where working.*	____	____
6. Lowered head of bed as low as possible to a level comfortable for client.*	____	____
7. Removed clothing from upper body.	____	____
8. Placed client on side or abdomen to expose entire back.	____	____
9. Put small amount of lotion on hands. Rubbed hands together to warm lotion.	____	____
10. Used correct body mechanics. Faced head of bed, one foot slightly forward, knees bent.	____	____
11. Started at the lower back and moved upward toward the shoulders. Applied pressure using palms of both hands. Used long, firm but gentle strokes: up, out, and down. Repeated several times.	____	____
12. Removed excess lotion with towel.	____	____
13. Helped client to put on clothes.	____	____
14. Made sure client was safe and comfortable.	____	____
15. Placed bed in lowest position. (Raised side rail, if indicated.)*	____	____
16. Washed hands.	____	____
17. Recorded what was done. Reported any unusual conditions to supervisor.	____	____

Comments:

Evaluator's Signature: _____

Date: _____

---

*Will not apply if hospital bed is not used.

PROCEDURE 14-8. GIVING PERINEAL CARE

Name: _____

	S	UN
1. Explained procedure to client.	___	___
2. Washed hands.	___	___
3. Obtained necessary materials.	___	___
4. Spread paper towel on work area. Arranged supplies on paper towel.	___	___
5. Provided privacy.	___	___
6. Raised bed to convenient working height. Lowered rail on side where working.*	___	___
7. Folded top bedding to foot of bed and covered client with sheet or blanket.	___	___
8. Helped client into supine position and removed clothing from waist down.	___	___
9. Positioned waterproof protector pad under buttocks.	___	___
10. Draped the client.	___	___
11. Raised side rail.*	___	___
12. Filled wash basin two-thirds full with warm water (105° to 110° F; 41° to 43° C).	___	___
13. Placed basin on work area on top of paper towels.	___	___
14. Lowered rail on side where work will be done.*	___	___
15. Folded back corner of blanket or sheet between client's legs and onto abdomen.	___	___
16. Helped client to bend knees and spread legs.	___	___
17. Put on disposable gloves.	___	___
18. Applied soap and water to washcloth or cotton balls.	___	___
19. Provided female perineal care:	___	___
a. Separated labia.	___	___
b. Cleaned downward, with one stroke, from front to back. Used clean washcloth or cotton ball for each stroke. Put used cotton balls in bag or set aside used washcloths. Repeated this step until area was clean.	___	___
c. Rinsed area, using same procedure as in steps 19a and 19b.	___	___
d. Dried area thoroughly.	___	___
e. Folded blanket back between client's legs.	___	___
f. Helped client to straighten legs and turn on side away from aide.	___	___
g. Separated buttocks and cleaned rectal area with toilet tissue, if needed. Washed area from vagina to anus, using clean washcloth for each stroke. Repeated this step until area was clean.	___	___
h. Rinsed area, using same procedure as in step 19g.	___	___
i. Dried area.	___	___

20. Provided male perineal care: ____ ____

   a. Gently pulled back foreskin if client is uncircumcised. ____ ____

   b. While holding penis, cleaned tip using a circular motion. Started at the urethral opening and worked outward. Repeated this step, using a clean washcloth or cotton ball, until area was clean. Put used cotton balls in bag or set aside used washcloths. ____ ____

   c. Rinsed and dried area thoroughly, using same procedure as steps 20a and 20b. ____ ____

   d. Returned foreskin to natural position if client is uncircumcised. ____ ____

   e. Cleaned shaft of penis using washcloth with firm but gentle downward strokes. Rinsed and dried area thoroughly. ____ ____

   f. Helped client to bend knees and spread legs. ____ ____

   g. Gently cleaned scrotum. Washed skin folds carefully. Rinsed and dried area thoroughly. ____ ____

   h. Helped client to straighten legs and turn on side away from aide. ____ ____

   i. Separated buttocks and cleaned rectal area with toilet tissue, if needed. Washed from scrotum to anus, using clean washcloth for each stroke. Repeated this step until area was clean. ____ ____

   j. Rinsed area using same procedure as in step 20i. ____ ____

   k. Dried area. ____ ____

21. Removed soiled bedding, washcloths, and waterproof protector pad and placed in laundry container. ____ ____

22. Removed gloves and discarded into bag. ____ ____

23. Straightened bedding; removed sheet or blanket. ____ ____

24. Made sure client was safe and comfortable. ____ ____

25. Placed bed in lowest position. (Raised side rail, if indicated.)* ____ ____

26. Emptied and cleaned washbasin. Wiped off work area with paper towels and discarded into bag. Returned other materials to their proper place. ____ ____

27. Washed hands. ____ ____

28. Recorded what was done. Reported any unusual conditions to supervisor. ____ ____

Comments:

Evaluator's Signature: _____

Date: _____

_____

*Will not apply if hospital bed is not used.

PROCEDURE 14-9. CARING FOR NAILS AND FEET

Name: _____

	S	**UN**
1. Explained procedure to client.	____	____
2. Washed hands.	____	____
3. Obtained necessary materials.	____	____
4. Spread paper towel on work area. Arranged supplies on paper towel.	____	____
5. Provided privacy.	____	____
6. Helped client into chair or to side of bed.	____	____
7. Assisted client to remove footwear, if appropriate.	____	____
8. Put bath mat, towel, or newspapers under feet.	____	____
9. Filled basin with warm water (100° to 110° F; 38° to 43° C).	____	____
10. Placed basin on bath mat. Put on gloves (optional). Helped client put feet in basin.	____	____
11. Allowed feet to soak for 10 minutes. Added warm water, as needed.	____	____
12. Placed table or ironing board in front of client at convenient height and close to client. Covered table with hand towel or paper towels.	____	____
13. Filled emesis basin or small bowl with warm water (100° to 110° F; 38° to 43° C). Put client's fingers in basin and soaked for 2 to 3 minutes.	____	____
14. Cleaned under fingernails with orangewood stick. Dried fingers thoroughly and set basin aside.	____	____
15. Shaped fingernails with emery board or nail file. Pushed back cuticles gently with washcloth or orangewood stick. Applied hand lotion (optional).	____	____
16. Removed table.	____	____
17. Removed one foot from basin. Smoothed any calloused areas using washcloth or pumice stone. Dried foot and between toes thoroughly. Repeated procedure for other foot. Applied lotion, as needed.	____	____
18. Removed gloves, if worn, and discarded.	____	____
19. Helped client to put on footwear or helped back to bed.	____	____
20. Cleaned equipment and stored in proper location. Discarded disposable supplies.	____	____
21. Placed soiled towels in laundry container to be washed.	____	____
22. Washed hands.	____	____
23. Recorded what was done. Reported any unusual conditions to supervisor.	____	____

Comments:

Evaluator's Signature: _____

Date: _____

PROCEDURE 14-10. ASSISTING CLIENT WITH HAIR CARE

Name: _____

	S	UN
1. Explained procedure to client.	____	____
2. Washed hands.	____	____
3. Obtained necessary materials.	____	____
4. Provided privacy.	____	____
5. Raised bed to convenient working height. Lowered rail on side of bed where aide is working.*	____	____
6. Placed client in upright position in bed or in chair, if possible.	____	____
7. Placed bath towel around client's shoulders. If client is in bed, placed towel under head to cover the pillow.	____	____
8. Parted hair and separated it into sections.	____	____
9. Brushed hair, section by section; worked from root to end of hair.	____	____
10. Arranged hair according to client's wishes.	____	____
11. Removed towel.	____	____
12. Made sure client was safe and comfortable.	____	____
13. Placed bed in lowest position.*	____	____
14. Cleaned supplies and stored in proper location.	____	____
15. Placed soiled bath towel in laundry container to be washed.	____	____
16. Washed hands.	____	____
17. Recorded what was done. Reported any unusual conditions to supervisor.	____	____

Comments:

Evaluator's Signature: _____

Date: _____

---

*Will not apply if hospital bed is not used.

PROCEDURE 14-11. GIVING A SHAMPOO

Name: _____

	S	UN
1. Explained procedure to client.	___	___
2. Washed hands.	___	___
3. Obtained necessary materials.	___	___
4. Provided privacy. Removed glasses and hearing aids, if needed. Stored properly.	___	___
5. Raised bed to convenient working height. Lowered rail on side of bed where aide is working.*	___	___
6. Positioned client for shampoo: at sink, in tub or shower, or in bed, with trough under head and neck.	___	___
7. Brushed and combed hair.	___	___
8. Had client hold folded washcloth over eyes to protect from shampoo.	___	___
9. Wet hair, from front to back, with warm water (100° F; 38° C).	___	___
10. Put a small amount of shampoo in palm of hand.	___	___
11. Applied shampoo to scalp; lathered from front to back, rubbing gently.	___	___
12. Rinsed thoroughly with warm water.	___	___
13. Repeated steps 10 through 12.	___	___
14. Applied conditioner, according to directions, and as desired by client.	___	___
15. Wrapped client's head in bath towel.	___	___
16. For bath or shower stall: helped client out. Assisted with drying body and hair.	___	___
17. For bed shampoo: removed trough from bed. Towel dried hair.	___	___
18. Dried hair using hair dryer, if available. Arranged hair according to client's wishes.	___	___
19. Made sure client was safe and comfortable. Replaced glasses and hearing aids, if appropriate.	___	___
20. Placed bed in lowest position. (Raised side rail, if indicated.)*	___	___
21. Cleaned materials and stored in proper location.	___	___
22. Placed soiled bath towel in laundry container.	___	___
23. Washed hands.	___	___
24. Recorded what was done. Reported any unusual conditions to supervisor.	___	___

Comments:

Evaluator's Signature: _____

Date: _____

---

*Will not apply if hospital bed is not used.

PROCEDURE 14-12. SHAVING THE MALE CLIENT

Name: _____

	S	UN
1. Explained procedure to client.	____	____
2. Washed hands.	____	____
3. Obtained necessary materials.	____	____
4. Provided privacy.	____	____
5. Raised bed to convenient working height. Lowered rail on side of bed where working.*	____	____
6. Placed client in an upright position in bed (or assisted to sit by bathroom sink, if possible).	____	____
7. Shaving with a blade razor:	____	____
a. Put on disposable gloves.	____	____
b. Wet washcloth with warm water (115° F; 46° C). Placed on client's face for a few minutes. Removed.	____	____
c. Applied shaving cream and lathered the face.	____	____
d. Held the skin taut and shaved in the direction of hair growth.	____	____
e. Rinsed razor blade when necessary.	____	____
f. Rinsed skin and dried with towel.	____	____
g. Assisted client to apply aftershave lotion (optional).	____	____
8. Shaving with an electric razor:	____	____
a. Put on disposable gloves.	____	____
b. Made sure face was clean and dry.	____	____
c. Turned on razor.	____	____
d. Held skin taut and shaved in the direction of hair growth.	____	____
e. Turned off razor.	____	____
f. Assisted client to apply aftershave lotion (optional).	____	____
9. Removed towel.	____	____
10. Removed and discarded gloves.	____	____
11. Made sure client was safe and comfortable.	____	____
12. Placed bed in lowest position. (Raised side rail if indicated.)*	____	____
13. Cleaned materials and stored in proper location.	____	____
14. Placed soiled linens in laundry container.	____	____
15. Washed hands.	____	____
16. Recorded what was done. Reported any unusual conditions to supervisor.	____	____

Comments: _____

Evaluator's Signature: _____

Date: _____

_____
*Will not apply if hospital bed is not used.

PROCEDURE 14-13. HELPING CLIENT TO DRESS

Name: _____

	S	UN

1. Explained procedure to client.   ____ ____

2. Washed hands.   ____ ____

3. Obtained necessary materials.   ____ ____

4. Arranged clothing in order of use.   ____ ____

5. Provided privacy.   ____ ____

6. Lowered bed to lowest position. Lowered rail on side where working.*   ____ ____

7. Helped client to sit on side of bed, if possible. If client must stay in bed, placed
   in supine position.   ____ ____

8. Helped client to put on undershirt or bra, shirt, or pajama top.   ____ ____

   a. Over-the-head type garment: placed injured arm into garment first.
      Pulled neck of garment over client's head. Guided other arm into garment.   ____ ____

   b. Front-button or zipping type garment: placed injured arm through sleeve first.
      Brought shirt to the back of client and guided the other arm into the sleeve.   ____ ____

9. Helped client to put on underwear, slacks, shorts, or pajama bottoms. If leg is
   injured, placed into garment first, then the other leg. Helped client to stand at side
   of bed and pulled up clothing to the waist. If client is in bed, helped client to lift buttocks
   and aide pulled up garments.   ____ ____

10. Helped client to put on socks or stockings and footwear.   ____ ____

11. Made sure client was safe and comfortable.   ____ ____

12. Placed bed in lowest position. (Raised side rail, if indicated).*   ____ ____

13. Washed hands.   ____ ____

14. Recorded what was done. Reported any unusual conditions to supervisor.   ____ ____

Comments:

Evaluator's Signature: _____

Date: _____

---

*Will not apply if hospital bed is not used.

PROCEDURE 14-14. HELPING CLIENT WITH AN INTRAVENOUS (IV) LINE TO REMOVE USED CLOTHING AND APPLY CLEAN CLOTHING

Name: _____

	S	UN
1. Explained procedure to client.	____	____
2. Washed hands.	____	____
3. Obtained necessary materials.	____	____
4. Arranged clothing in order of use.	____	____
5. Provided privacy.	____	____
6. Lowered bed to lowest position. Lowered rail on side of bed.*	____	____
7. Helped client to sit on side of bed, if possible. If client must stay in bed, placed in supine position.	____	____
8. Helped client to remove used garment from arm without IV.	____	____
9. Gathered up sleeve of garment on arm with IV. Slid sleeve over IV site and tubing. Removed client's arm and hand from sleeve.	____	____
10. Slid hand along tubing to IV bag, keeping sleeve gathered.	____	____
11. Removed IV from pole. Slid bag and tubing through sleeve. Kept bag above client's arm. Did not pull on tubing. Placed used clothing on chair.	____	____
12. Hung IV bag back on pole.	____	____
13. Gathered sleeve of clean garment to be put on arm with IV.	____	____
14. Removed IV bag from pole. Made sure bag was above client's arm.	____	____
15. Slipped sleeve and garment shoulder over IV bag. Placed bag back on pole.	____	____
16. Slid gathered sleeve over the tubing, hand, arm, and IV site.	____	____
17. Adjusted garment over client's shoulders and helped client to put other arm through other sleeve.	____	____
18. Checked that IV was working properly.	____	____
19. Assisted client to remove other garments and put on clean garments, as needed.	____	____
20. Made sure client was safe and comfortable.	____	____
21. Placed soiled garments in laundry container.	____	____
22. Placed bed in lowest position. (Raised side rail, if indicated.)*	____	____
23. Recorded what was done. Reported any unusual conditions to supervisor.	____	____

Comments:

Evaluator's Signature: _____

Date: _____

_____
*Will not apply if hospital bed is not used.

PROCEDURE 14-15. HELPING WITH RANGE-OF-MOTION EXERCISES IN BED: GENERAL PROCEDURE

Name: _____

	S	**UN**
1. Explained procedure to client.	___	___
2. Washed hands.	___	___
3. Provided privacy.	___	___
4. Raised bed to convenient working height. Lowered rail on side of bed where working.*	___	___
5. Folded top bedding to foot of bed. Covered client with sheet or blanket.	___	___
6. Helped client to move to side of bed near aide. Made sure client was in supine position.	___	___
7. Repeated each exercise as listed in the care plan.	___	___
8. Exercised upper body, both sides. Then exercised lower body, both sides.	___	___
9. Helped client to center of bed. Replaced top bedding, and removed sheet or blanket covering client.	___	___
10. Made sure client was safe and comfortable.	___	___
11. Placed bed in lowest position. (Raised side rail, if indicated.)*	___	___
12. Washed hands.	___	___
13. Recorded what was done. Reported any unusual conditions to supervisor or physical therapist.	___	___

Shoulder and Arm Exercises

Held client's wrist and hand with one hand. With other hand, grasped client's arm above elbow.	___	___
a. Moved arm, with palm down, forward and upward along side of client's head and then downward to the side. Repeated with palm up.	___	___
b. Moved arm, with palm down, away from the body, sideways, to above the head, and returned. Repeated with palm up.	___	___

Forearm and Elbow Exercises

Rested client's upper arm on bed, with forearm raised upright and elbow bent. Supported client's wrist and hand.	___	___
a. Moved lower arm down, then up, with palm down. Repeated with palm up.	___	___
Rested client's upper arm on bed with forearm upright. Supported client's wrist with one hand and client's hand with the other.	___	___
a. Turned palm toward client, then away.	___	___

Wrist Exercises

Held client's wrist with one hand and used other hand to perform movements:	___	___
a. Moved hand forward, then backward.	___	___
b. Moved hand from one side to the other.	___	___

Finger Exercises

Held client's wrist with one hand and used other hand to perform movements:	___	___
a. Bent fingers (made a fist), then straightened.	___	___
b. Spread fingers and thumb apart, then brought together.	___	___

Thumb Exercises

Held client's hand and fingers with one hand. Used other hand to perform movements: ____ ____

    a. Moved thumb across palm of hand and straightened, then returned to side.   ____ ____

    b. Touched each fingertip with thumb.   ____ ____

    c. Bent thumb into palm and returned to straightened position.   ____ ____

    d. Moved thumb using a wide, circular motion.   ____ ____

Hip, Leg, and Knee Exercises

Supported client's leg with one hand under knee and other at the heel.   ____ ____

    a. Bent knee and raised toward chest, then lowered.   ____ ____

    b. Raised leg straight up as high as possible, then lowered leg gently.   ____ ____

Supported client's leg with one hand under knee and other hand under ankle.   ____ ____

    a. Moved leg outward, away from body as far as possible. Returned to starting position.   ____ ____

    b. Moved leg across other leg as far as possible, then returned to starting position.   ____ ____

Placed one hand over top of knee and grasped. Placed other hand over top of ankle and grasped.   ____ ____

    a. Turned leg so toes pointed inward, then outward.   ____ ____

Supported client's leg with one hand just above the knee and the other hand at the ankle.   ____ ____

    a. Bent the knee and slid the heel toward the buttocks as far as possible. Then straightened knee to starting position.   ____ ____

Foot and Ankle Exercises

Supported ankle by placing client's heel in palm of one hand, with other hand just above the ankle.   ____ ____

    a. Bent foot up toward the leg, then down, away from leg.   ____ ____

    b. Turned foot outward, sole facing away from body, then turned foot inward toward body.   ____ ____

Toe Exercises

Held client's foot with one hand. Used other hand to perform movements: ____ ____

    a. Bent toes down toward the ball of the foot, then bent toes back to front of foot.   ____ ____

Comments:

Evaluator's Signature: _____

Date: _____

---

*Will not apply if hospital bed is not used.

PROCEDURE 15-1. GIVING AND REMOVING A BEDPAN

Name: _____

	S	UN
1. Explained procedure to client.	___	___
2. Washed hands.	___	___
3. Obtained necessary materials.	___	___
4. Provided privacy.	___	___
5. Raised bed to convenient working height.*	___	___
6. Warmed bedpan with warm tap water. Dried with paper towels.	___	___
7. Took bedpan to bedside and placed on chair or bed.	___	___
8. Lowered side rail.*	___	___
9. Assisted client to lie on back. Elevated head of bed slightly.*	___	___
10. Folded back upper linens.	___	___
11. Instructed client to bend knees and raise buttocks. Assisted as needed. If bed or client was soiled, put on gloves.	___	___
12. Slid bedpan under client.	___	___
13. If client could not raise hips to get onto bedpan, aide:	___	___
a. Turned client on side, facing away from aide.	___	___
b. Positioned bedpan firmly against client's buttocks.	___	___
c. Turned client onto back and held the bedpan in place under the buttocks.	___	___
14. Covered client with top sheet.	___	___
15. Raised side rail and placed bed in sitting position.*	___	___
16. Propped up client with pillows if bed not adjustable.	___	___
17. Made sure bedpan was in correct position.	___	___
18. Gave toilet tissue and asked client to call when finished.	___	___
19. Left room. Removed gloves, if using. Discarded gloves.	___	___
20. Washed hands.	___	___
21. Returned to room when client called.	___	___
22. Lowered rail on side where working.*	___	___
23. Put on gloves.	___	___
24. Placed client in flat position and removed bedpan in same manner used to give bedpan.	___	___
25. Cleansed perineal area with toilet tissue, if necessary, wiping from front to back.	___	___
26. Raised side rail.*	___	___
27. Covered bedpan, took to bathroom, and emptied contents. Measured output, if necessary. Observed contents.	___	___
28. Rinsed bedpan with cold water, cleaned, and disinfected.	___	___

29. Removed and discarded gloves.   ____ ____

30. Washed hands.   ____ ____

31. Put bedpan away.   ____ ____

32. Lowered rail on side where working.*   ____ ____

33. Helped client to wash hands.   ____ ____

34. Made sure client was safe and comfortable.   ____ ____

35. Placed bed in lowest position. (Raised side rail, if indicated.)*   ____ ____

36. Washed hands.   ____ ____

37. Recorded what was done. Reported any unusual elimination to supervisor.   ____ ____

Comments:

Evaluator's Signature: _____

Date: _____

---

*Will not apply if hospital bed is not used.

PROCEDURE 15-2. GIVING AND REMOVING A URINAL

Name: _____

	S	UN
1. Explained procedure to client	____	____
2. Washed hands.	____	____
3. Obtained necessary materials.	____	____
4. Provided privacy.	____	____
5. Took urinal to bedside and placed on chair or bed.	____	____
6. Assisted client to stand. If client could not stand, placed client on back.	____	____
7. Folded back upper linens.	____	____
8. Gave urinal to client so he could position it properly.	____	____
9. If client was unable to position urinal, put on gloves and positioned it for him.	____	____
10. Covered client with top sheet.	____	____
11. Left room. Removed gloves, if used. Discarded gloves.	____	____
12. Washed hands.	____	____
13. Returned to room when client called.	____	____
14. Put on gloves.	____	____
15. Removed urinal in the same manner it was given.	____	____
16. Covered urinal, took to bathroom, and emptied contents. Measured output, if necessary. Observed urine.	____	____
17. Rinsed urinal with cold water, cleaned, and disinfected.	____	____
18. Removed and discarded gloves.	____	____
19. Washed hands.	____	____
20. Put urinal away.	____	____
21. Helped client to wash hands.	____	____
22. Made sure client was safe and comfortable.	____	____
23. Washed hands.	____	____
24. Recorded what was done. Reported any unusual urine or urination to supervisor.	____	____

Comments:

Evaluator's Signature: _____

Date: _____

PROCEDURE 15-3. MEASURING AND RECORDING INTAKE AND OUTPUT

Name: _____

Intake	**S**	**UN**
1. Washed hands.	____	____
2. Obtained necessary materials.	____	____
3. Measured each remaining liquid separately after client finished eating or drinking. Poured into measuring cup.	____	____
4. Held at eye level and measured amount left.	____	____
5. Subtracted remaining amount from amount of the original full serving.	____	____
6. Repeated for each liquid and recorded.	____	____
7. Rinsed, cleaned, dried, and stored container used to measure intake.	____	____
8. Washed hands.	____	____
9. Accurately recorded amount of fluid intake and the time on the I&O form.	____	____

Output		
1. Washed hands.	____	____
2. Put on gloves and other personal protective equipment, as needed.	____	____
3. Emptied bedpan, urinal, commode pail, "hat," or emesis basin into graduated container if original container not marked for measuring.	____	____
4. Measured amount of liquid and discarded into toilet.	____	____
5. Rinsed, cleaned, disinfected, dried, and stored container used to measure output.	____	____
6. Removed and discarded gloves and other personal protective equipment.	____	____
7. Washed hands.	____	____
8. Accurately recorded amount of fluid output and the time on the I&O form.	____	____
9. Reported any unusual output to supervisor.	____	____

Comments:

Evaluator's Signature: _____

Date: _____

PROCEDURE 15-4. CARE OF THE CLIENT WITH AN INDWELLING CATHETER

Name: _____

	S	UN

1. Explained procedure to client. ____ ____

2. Washed hands. ____ ____

3. Obtained necessary materials. ____ ____

4. Provided privacy. ____ ____

5. Put on gloves. ____ ____

6. Performed perineal care. ____ ____

7. Female client: Separated labia to visualize the urinary meatus. Male client: Retracted foreskin (if uncircumcised). ____ ____

8. Moistened cotton balls or gauze with soap and water. ____ ____

9. Washed catheter tube in a downward motion away from urinary meatus for approximately 4 inches (20 cm). Used one cotton ball or gauze pad for each stroke. Rinsed with water in same manner. Discarded used cotton balls or gauze into bag. ____ ____

10. Taped and positioned catheter properly. ____ ____

11. Removed waterproof protector pad. Replaced top linens. ____ ____

12. Made sure client was safe and comfortable. ____ ____

13. Cleaned materials and stored in proper location. ____ ____

14. Removed and discarded gloves. ____ ____

15. Washed hands. ____ ____

16. Recorded what was done. Reported any unusual conditions to supervisor. ____ ____

Comments:

Evaluator's Signature: _____

Date: _____

PROCEDURE 15-5. EMPTYING A CATHETER DRAINAGE BAG

Name: _____

	S	UN
1. Explained procedure to client.	____	____
2. Washed hands.	____	____
3. Obtained necessary materials.	____	____
4. Provided privacy.	____	____
5. Put on gloves and other personal protective equipment, as needed.	____	____
6. Placed measuring container under drainage tube of collection bag.	____	____
7. Opened clamp on drainage tube so urine could empty into graduate. Drainage tube did not touch insides of graduated container or any other surface.	____	____
8. Closed clamp and replaced drainage tube in the holder on collection bag.	____	____
9. Measured urine, then discarded in toilet.	____	____
10. Rinsed, cleaned, disinfected, and stored graduate.	____	____
11. Removed and discarded gloves and other personal protective equipment.	____	____
12. Washed hands.	____	____
13. Recorded what was done. Reported any unusual conditions to supervisor.	____	____

Comments:

Evaluator's Signature: _____

Date: _____

PROCEDURE 15-6. APPLYING A CONDOM CATHETER

Name: _____

	S	UN
1. Explained procedure to client.	___	___
2. Washed hands.	___	___
3. Obtained necessary materials.	___	___
4. Provided privacy.	___	___
5. Helped client to lie on back.	___	___
6. Put on gloves.	___	___
7. Covered client with sheet or bath blanket, as for perineal care.	___	___
8. If condom catheter was present, removed gently and placed in plastic bag.	___	___
9. Provided perineal care.	___	___
10. Attached collection bag to leg or bed frame.	___	___
11. Applied protective coating to skin of the penis if a self-adhesive catheter was used.	___	___
12. Held penis firmly. Rolled condom catheter onto penis, with drainage opening at the urinary meatus.	___	___
13. Secured edge of condom catheter in place with Velcro band. Was careful not to constrict the penis.	___	___
14. Connected catheter tip to drainage tubing.	___	___
15. Made sure tubing was in correct position and that tip of catheter was not twisted.	___	___
16. Made sure client was safe and comfortable.	___	___
17. Discarded used supplies in plastic bag.	___	___
18. Removed and discarded gloves.	___	___
19. Washed hands.	___	___
20. Recorded what was done. Reported any unusual findings to supervisor.	___	___

Comments:

Evaluator's Signature: _____

Date: _____

PROCEDURE 16-1. COLLECTING A ROUTINE URINE SPECIMEN

Name: _____

	S	UN
1. Explained procedure to client.	___	___
2. Washed hands.	___	___
3. Obtained necessary materials.	___	___
4. Labeled container and placed in bathroom.	___	___
5. Put on gloves and other personal protective equipment, as needed.	___	___
6. Assisted client to bathroom or commode or offered bedpan or urinal.	___	___
7. Reminded client not to drop toilet tissue into specimen. Asked client to discard toilet tissue into waste basket.	___	___
8. Had client void into commode, bedpan, urinal, or "hat."	___	___
9. Took bedpan, urinal, or commode pail into bathroom.	___	___
10. Poured urine into graduate and then into specimen container until three-fourths full. Discarded remaining urine into toilet.	___	___
11. Put lid on specimen container.	___	___
12. Placed container into a plastic bag and then into paper bag.	___	___
13. Cleaned materials and stored in proper location.	___	___
14. Removed and discarded gloves and other personal protective equipment.	___	___
15. Washed hands.	___	___
16. Helped client, as needed, back to bed or chair.	___	___
17. Stored specimen in refrigerator.	___	___
18. Recorded what was done. Reported any unusual conditions to supervisor.	___	___

Comments:

Evaluator's Signature: _____

Date: _____

PROCEDURE 16-2. COLLECTING A "CLEAN CATCH" OR MIDSTREAM URINE SPECIMEN

Name: _____

	S	UN
1. Explained procedure to client.	___	___
2. Washed hands.	___	___
3. Obtained necessary materials.	___	___
4. Opened kit. Removed contents and labeled container.	___	___
5. Assisted client to bathroom or commode, or offered bedpan or urinal.	___	___
6. Told client how to perform procedure. Instructed client to call when finished.	___	___
7. If assistance was necessary, put on gloves.	___	___
8. Provided perineal care using towelettes in specimen kit.	___	___
9. Kept client's labia separated until specimen was collected so that urine did not flow over skin surfaces. In uncircumcised males, the foreskin was retracted until the specimen was collected.	___	___
10. Collected the specimen:	___	___
a. Asked client to begin voiding into urinal, bedpan, commode, or toilet.	___	___
b. Instructed client to stop voiding.	___	___
c. Held specimen container under urinary meatus but did not allow it to touch skin surface. Did not touch inside of container with hands.	___	___
d. Asked client to restart voiding.	___	___
e. Caught enough urine to fill container about halfway.	___	___
f. Asked client to stop voiding.	___	___
g. Removed container.	___	___
h. Instructed client to finish voiding.	___	___
11. Put lid on specimen container. Was careful not to touch inside to keep the specimen clean.	___	___
12. Placed container into a plastic bag and then into a paper bag.	___	___
13. Assisted client to complete toileting, if necessary.	___	___
14. Cleaned materials and stored in proper location.	___	___
15. Removed and discarded gloves.	___	___
16. Washed hands.	___	___
17. Helped client, as needed, back to bed or chair.	___	___
18. Stored specimen in refrigerator.	___	___
19. Recorded what was done. Reported any unusual conditions to supervisor.	___	___

Comments:

Evaluator's Signature: _____

Date: _____

PROCEDURE 16-3. COLLECTING A 24-HOUR URINE SPECIMEN

Name: _____

	S	UN
1. Explained procedure to client and family.	___	___
2. Washed hands.	___	___
3. Obtained necessary materials.	___	___
4. Labeled container.	___	___
5. Arranged urine container in bucket of ice in bathroom. Placed preservative in container, if needed.	___	___
6. Placed sign saying "Save All Urine" in bathroom near toilet.	___	___
7. Put on gloves and other personal protective equipment, as needed.	___	___
8. Had client void first specimen. Discarded. Recorded time.	___	___
9. Removed and discarded gloves and other personal protective equipment after first specimen and each time another specimen was handled. Discarded gloves and other personal protective equipment. Washed hands.	___	___
10. Collected all urine for next 24 hours. Poured into specimen container.	___	___
11. Reminded client not to have a bowel movement when urinating.	___	___
12. Recorded I&O, if needed.	___	___
13. Added each urine specimen to the container immediately after voiding. Poured into graduate using funnel, if needed, and then into large container to avoid spilling and splashing.	___	___
14. Added ice to bucket, as necessary.	___	___
15. At end of 24 hours, had client void as before. Placed final specimen in large container.	___	___
16. Recorded what was done. Reported any problems or unusual conditions to supervisor.	___	___
17. Kept specimen on ice.	___	___
18. Dried container and placed it in large plastic grocery bag for delivery to laboratory.	___	___

Comments:

Evaluator's Signature: _____

Date: _____

PROCEDURE 16-4. STRAINING URINE

Name: _____

	S	UN
1. Explained procedure to client and family.	___	___
2. Obtained necessary materials and placed in bathroom.	___	___
3. Placed sign saying "Strain All Urine" near toilet.	___	___
4. Washed hands.	___	___
5. Put on gloves (and goggles, if needed).	___	___
6. Had client void into bedpan, urinal, commode, or urine collector (hat) in toilet.	___	___
7. Transferred urine into graduated container.	___	___
8. Placed strainer or gauze over specimen container.	___	___
9. Poured urine through strainer and into specimen container.	___	___
10. Inspected filter paper or gauze. If stones present, wrapped them in filter material and placed in the specimen container for transport to laboratory. Labeled container. Stored in refrigerator.	___	___
11. If no stones were present, discarded urine. Discarded used disposable materials. Cleaned used reusable materials and prepared for reuse next time client voids.	___	___
12. Removed and discarded gloves. Removed goggles, if used.	___	___
13. Washed hands.	___	___
14. Recorded what was done. Reported any unusual conditions to supervisor.	___	___

Comments:

Evaluator's Signature: _____

Date: _____

PROCEDURE 16-5. COLLECTING A STOOL SPECIMEN

Name: _____

	S	UN
1. Explained procedure to client.	____	____
2. Washed hands.	____	____
3. Obtained necessary materials.	____	____
4. Labeled container.	____	____
5. Assisted client to bathroom or commode or offered bedpan.	____	____
6. Asked client not to urinate, if possible, while having bowel movement.	____	____
7. Put on gloves.	____	____
8. Transferred stool specimen to container using tongue depressor or disposable spoon and put on lid.	____	____
9. Flushed remaining feces down toilet and assisted client to complete toileting, as necessary.	____	____
10. Removed and discarded gloves.	____	____
11. Washed hands.	____	____
12. Helped client, as needed, back to bed, chair, etc.	____	____
13. Stored specimen according to agency policy or supervisor's instructions.	____	____
14. Recorded what was done. Reported any unusual conditions to supervisor.	____	____

Comments:

Evaluator's Signature: _____

Date: _____

PROCEDURE 16-6. COLLECTING A SPUTUM SPECIMEN

Name: _____

	S	UN
1. Explained procedure to client.	___	___
2. Washed hands.	___	___
3. Obtained necessary materials.	___	___
4. Labeled container.	___	___
5. Provided privacy.	___	___
6. Put on gloves (disposable mask, if needed).	___	___
7. Assisted client to rinse mouth with plain water.	___	___
8. Had client hold sputum specimen container in one hand and tissue in the other.	___	___
9. Instructed client to take a deep breath, hold it for a second, and then cough into tissue. Did not let client cough on aide. Had client repeat the coughing two or three times to loosen sputum deep in the respiratory tract.	___	___
10. When client had loosened sputum, had client cough sputum directly into the specimen container.	___	___
11. Did not touch inside of the container. Kept outside of container clean and free of any sputum.	___	___
12. Put lid on specimen container.	___	___
13. Placed container into plastic bag and then into a paper bag.	___	___
14. Removed and discarded gloves (removed and discarded mask if worn).	___	___
15. Washed hands.	___	___
16. Recorded what was done. Reported any unusual conditions to supervisor.	___	___
17. Sent specimen to laboratory according to agency policy.	___	___

Comments:

Evaluator's Signature: _____

Date: _____

PROCEDURE 17-1. CLEANING A THERMOMETER

Name: _____

	S	UN
1. Washed hands.	___	___
2. Obtained necessary materials.	___	___
3. Put on disposable gloves.	___	___
4. Wet cotton ball (or tissue) with soap and water.	___	___
5. Held thermometer by stem over sink or wastebasket.	___	___
6. Began at stem end. Washed from stem to bulb end, twisting cotton ball firmly.	___	___
7. Discarded used cotton ball.	___	___
8. Rinsed thermometer with a clean, wet cotton ball using the same twisting, downward movement.	___	___
9. Repeated washing and rinsing.	___	___
10. Dried with a tissue, wiping in the same downward movement.	___	___
11. Discarded tissue.	___	___
12. Stored thermometer properly.	___	___
13. Removed and discarded gloves. Washed hands.	___	___

Comments:

Evaluator's Signature: _____

Date: _____

PROCEDURE 17-2. TAKING AN ORAL TEMPERATURE (WITH A REGULAR THERMOMETER)

Name: _____

	S	**UN**
1. Explained procedure to client. Reminded client not to eat, drink, or smoke for 15 minutes.	____	____
2. Had client lie down or rest in a chair.	____	____
3. Washed hands.	____	____
4. Obtained necessary materials.	____	____
5. Put on disposable gloves (optional).	____	____
6. Cleaned thermometer.	____	____
7. Shook down thermometer to 95° F (35° C), if necessary.	____	____
8. Placed thermometer under client's tongue, as far back as possible, into either heat pocket.	____	____
9. Told client to keep mouth closed and not to talk.	____	____
10. Left thermometer in place for 3 minutes. Took client's pulse and respirations at this time.	____	____
11. Removed thermometer.	____	____
12. Wiped thermometer with tissue from stem end to bulb end. Discarded tissue. Did not touch any part of thermometer that had been in client's mouth.	____	____
13. Read thermometer and then placed it on a tissue.	____	____
14. Wrote the temperature (pulse and respirations) on the paper.	____	____
15. Cleaned and dried thermometer.	____	____
16. Shook down thermometer to 95° F (35° C).	____	____
17. Stored thermometer in holder in proper location.	____	____
18. Removed and discarded gloves (optional). Washed hands.	____	____
19. Recorded temperature on client record. Indicated (O) for oral temperature.	____	____
20. Reported any abnormal temperature to supervisor.	____	____

Comments:

Evaluator's Signature: _____

Date: _____

PROCEDURE 17-3. TAKING AN ORAL TEMPERATURE (WITH AN ELECTRONIC THERMOMETER)

Name: _____

	S	UN
1. Explained procedure to client. Reminded client not to eat, drink, or smoke for 15 minutes.	___	___
2. Had client lie down or rest in a chair.	___	___
3. Washed hands.	___	___
4. Obtained necessary materials.	___	___
5. Put on disposable gloves (optional).	___	___
6. Cleaned thermometer.	___	___
7. Turned on thermometer.	___	___
8. Waited until thermometer read "0" or showed "- - -" on the digital display window.	___	___
9. Placed thermometer under client's tongue, as far back as possible, into either heat pocket.	___	___
10. Told client to keep mouth closed and not to talk.	___	___
11. Left thermometer in place until it beeped. Took client's pulse and respirations at this time.	___	___
12. Removed thermometer.	___	___
13. Wiped thermometer with tissue from stem end to bulb end. Discarded tissue. Did not touch any part of thermometer that had been in client's mouth.	___	___
14. Read thermometer and then placed it on a tissue.	___	___
15. Wrote the temperature (pulse and respirations) on the paper.	___	___
16. Cleaned and dried thermometer.	___	___
17. Turned off thermometer.	___	___
18. Stored thermometer in holder in proper location.	___	___
19. Removed and discarded gloves (optional). Washed hands.	___	___
20. Recorded temperature on client record. Indicated (O) for oral temperature.	___	___
21. Reported abnormal temperature to supervisor.	___	___

Comments:

Evaluator's Signature: _____

Date: _____

PROCEDURE 17-4. TAKING AN ORAL TEMPERATURE (WITH A SINGLE-USE THERMOMETER)

Name: _____

	S	UN
1. Explained procedure to client. Reminded client not to eat, drink, or smoke for 15 minutes.	____	____
2. Had client lie down or rest in a chair.	____	____
3. Washed hands.	____	____
4. Obtained necessary materials.	____	____
5. Removed thermometer from wrapper.	____	____
6. Placed thermometer under client's tongue, as far back as possible, into either heat pocket.	____	____
7. Told client to keep mouth closed and not to talk.	____	____
8. Left thermometer in place for at least 1 minute. Took client's pulse and respirations at this time.	____	____
9. Removed thermometer. Did not touch any part of thermometer that had been in client's mouth. Waited 10 seconds and read the last colored dot on the thermometer. Placed the thermometer on a tissue.	____	____
10. Wrote the client's temperature, pulse, and respirations on the paper.	____	____
11. Discarded thermometer.	____	____
12. Washed hands.	____	____
13. Recorded temperature on client record. Indicated (O) for oral temperature.	____	____
14. Reported abnormal temperature to supervisor.	____	____

Comments:

Evaluator's Signature: _____

Date: _____

PROCEDURE 17-5. TAKING AN AXILLARY TEMPERATURE

Name: _____

	S	UN
1. Explained procedure to client.	____	____
2. Had client lie down or sit down.	____	____
3. Washed hands.	____	____
4. Obtained necessary materials.	____	____
5. Cleaned thermometer.	____	____
6. Shook down thermometer to 95° F (35° C), turned on electronic thermometer, or removed single-use thermometer from wrapper.	____	____
7. Provided privacy.	____	____
8. Removed client's arm from sleeve. Exposed axilla.	____	____
9. Dried axilla with towel or washcloth.	____	____
10. Placed thermometer in axilla so that it was in contact with skin. Put client's arm across chest to hold thermometer in place. For infant or child, held arm in place, as necessary.	____	____
11. Left thermometer in place:	____	____
a. Regular thermometer: 10 minutes	____	____
b. Electronic thermometer: until a beep was heard	____	____
c. Single-use thermometer: 3 minutes	____	____
Took client's pulse and respirations at this time.	____	____
12. Removed thermometer.	____	____
13. Wiped with tissue from stem end to bulb. Discarded tissue.	____	____
14. Read thermometer and then placed it on a tissue.	____	____
15. Wrote the temperature on the paper.	____	____
16. Helped client put arm back in sleeve.	____	____
17. Turned off electronic thermometer, if used.	____	____
18. Cleaned and dried thermometer. Or discarded single-use thermometer.	____	____
19. Shook down regular thermometer, if used.	____	____
20. Stored thermometer in holder in proper location.	____	____
21. Washed hands.	____	____
22. Recorded temperature on client record. Indicated (A) for axillary temperature.	____	____
23. Reported abnormal temperature to supervisor.	____	____

Comments:

Evaluator's Signature: _____

Date: _____

PROCEDURE 17-6. TAKING A TEMPERATURE USING A TYMPANIC THERMOMETER

Name: _____

	S	UN
1. Explained procedure to client.	___	___
2. Had client lie down or rest in a chair.	___	___
3. Provided privacy.	___	___
4. Washed hands.	___	___
5. Obtained necessary materials.	___	___
6. Asked client to turn head so ear was in front of aide.	___	___
7. Pulled top of ear up and back to straighten the ear canal in adults, or pulled earlobe down and back for children younger than 2 years of age.	___	___
8. Gently inserted tympanic thermometer probe with cover into the ear canal.	___	___
9. Read temperature measurement when flashing light was seen or tone heard.	___	___
10. Removed thermometer probe from ear canal.	___	___
11. Discarded probe cover directly into wastebasket.	___	___
12. Wrote the temperature on the paper. Indicated (T) for tympanic temperature.	___	___
13. Returned thermometer to base unit for recharge.	___	___
14. Washed hands.	___	___
15. Recorded what was done. Reported abnormal temperature to supervisor.	___	___

Comments:

Evaluator's Signature: _____

Date: _____

PROCEDURE 17-7. TAKING A RECTAL TEMPERATURE

Name: _____

	S	UN
1. Explained procedure to client.	____	____
2. Put client in bed.	____	____
3. Washed hands.	____	____
4. Obtained necessary materials.	____	____
5. Cleaned thermometer.	____	____
6. Shook down thermometer to 95° F (35° C), if necessary.	____	____
7. Provided privacy.	____	____
8. Placed client in Sims' position.	____	____
9. Put on gloves.	____	____
10. Placed small amount of lubricant on toilet tissue. Lubricated bulb end of thermometer.	____	____
11. Folded back top linens and removed clothing to expose anal area.	____	____
12. Raised upper buttock to expose anal area.	____	____
13. Gently inserted thermometer 1 inch (2.5 cm) into the rectum.	____	____
14. Held in place for 3 minutes.	____	____
15. Removed thermometer.	____	____
16. Wiped thermometer with toilet tissue from stem end to bulb end. Placed soiled tissue on several folded layers of toilet tissue.	____	____
17. Placed thermometer on clean toilet tissue.	____	____
18. Cleansed excess lubricant and feces from anal area using toilet tissue.	____	____
19. Replaced client's clothing and covered client.	____	____
20. Discarded soiled toilet tissue into toilet.	____	____
21. Removed and discarded gloves. Washed hands.	____	____
22. Read thermometer and then placed it back on tissue.	____	____
23. Wrote the temperature on the paper.	____	____
24. Cleaned and dried thermometer. Discarded single-use thermometer.	____	____
25. Shook down regular thermometer to 95° F (35° C).	____	____
26. Stored thermometer in holder in proper location.	____	____
27. Washed hands.	____	____
28. Made sure client was safe and comfortable.	____	____
29. Recorded temperature on client record. Indicated (R) for rectal temperature.	____	____
30. Reported abnormal temperature to supervisor.	____	____

Comments:

Evaluator's Signature: _____

Date: _____

PROCEDURE 17-8. TAKING A RADIAL PULSE

Name: _____

	S	UN
1. Explained procedure to client.	____	____
2. Asked client to sit or lie down.	____	____
3. Washed hands.	____	____
4. Obtained necessary materials.	____	____
5. Located radial pulse. Used middle three fingers to press down on client's radial artery.	____	____
6. Noted the following:	____	____
• Strong or weak	____	____
• Regular or irregular	____	____
7. Counted beats for 1 minute.	____	____
8. Wrote the pulse rate on the paper. Also noted the strength and regularity of beats.	____	____
9. Made sure client was safe and comfortable.	____	____
10. Recorded pulse on client record.	____	____
11. Reported any abnormal pulse conditions to supervisor.	____	____

Comments:

Evaluator's Signature: _____

Date: _____

PROCEDURE 17-9. TAKING RESPIRATIONS

Name: _____

	S	UN
1. Continued holding client's wrist after taking the pulse.	____	____
2. Did not tell client that respirations were going to be counted.	____	____
3. Counted each rise and fall of client's chest or abdomen as one respiration.	____	____
4. Counted respirations for 1 minute.	____	____
5. Observed for the following:	____	____
• Deep or shallow breathing	____	____
• Painful or difficulty breathing	____	____
• Noisy breathing	____	____
6. Recorded the respirations on the paper, noting the information listed above.	____	____
7. Made sure client was safe and comfortable.	____	____
8. Washed hands.	____	____
9. Recorded respirations on client record.	____	____
10. Reported any abnormal respirations to supervisor.	____	____

Comments:

Evaluator's Signature: _____

Date: _____

PROCEDURE 17-10. MEASURING BLOOD PRESSURE

Name: _____

	S	UN
1. Explained procedure to client.	____	____
2. Asked client to sit or lie down.	____	____
3. Washed hands.	____	____
4. Obtained necessary materials.	____	____
5. Wiped stethoscope earpieces and chestpiece (diaphragm) or bell with antiseptic wipes.	____	____
6. Placed client's arm in position level with the heart, palm up, and supported by a pillow, a table, or an arm of a chair.	____	____
7. Exposed client's upper arm. Removed clothing so that area was bare.	____	____
8. Squeezed blood pressure cuff to expel any air. Closed the valve of the bulb.	____	____
9. Found the brachial artery by feeling the pulse at the inner side of the elbow.	____	____
10. Wrapped the cuff around the client's arm, at least 1 inch above the bend in the arm. Made sure cuff was secure and even. Positioned rubber bag over the artery.	____	____
11. Put stethoscope earpieces in ears.	____	____
12. Placed fingers over radial pulse. Inflated the cuff until radial pulse could not be felt. Inflated cuff 30 mm beyond point at which pulse was last felt.	____	____
13. Placed stethoscope chestpiece (diaphragm) or bell over the brachial artery.	____	____
14. Kept eyes on dial and began to deflate cuff slowly and evenly (2 to 4 mm per second) by turning the valve of the bulb counterclockwise.	____	____
15. Noted the first sound heard and read the dial at that point.	____	____
16. Kept eyes on dial and continued to deflate the cuff. Noted the last sound heard and read the dial at that point.	____	____
17. Deflated cuff completely. Removed stethoscope and cuff from client's arm.	____	____
18. Wrote the blood pressure measurement on the paper.	____	____
19. Assisted client, as needed, to desired position.	____	____
20. Cleaned earpieces and chestpiece (diaphragm) or bell of stethoscope with antiseptic wipes. Discarded used wipes.	____	____
21. Returned all materials to proper storage place.	____	____
22. Washed hands.	____	____
23. Recorded accurate blood pressure on client record.	____	____
24. Reported blood pressure that was above or below normal to supervisor.	____	____

Comments:

Evaluator's Signature: _____

Date: _____

PROCEDURE 18-1. ASSISTING WITH ORAL MEDICATIONS

Name: _____

	S	UN
1. Explained procedure to client.	____	____
2. Checked care plan and medication sheet.	____	____
3. Washed hands.	____	____
4. Obtained necessary materials.	____	____
5. Helped client to wash hands.	____	____
6. Checked label on each presecription or on each prepoured medication for the following:	____	____
• Right drug	____	____
• Right client	____	____
• Right dose	____	____
• Right route	____	____
• Right time	____	____
7. Loosened lid(s) on container(s) if client was unable to do so. Told client name of each medication (read from label).	____	____
8. Placed containers where client could reach them or handed containers to client. Let client read name of medication to aide. Made sure client was wearing eyeglasses, if needed.	____	____
9. Assisted client with oral medications:	____	____
a. Gave sip of water to moisten mouth.	____	____
b. Supported hand as necessary to pour medication.	____	____
c. Gave client full glass of water or other cool liquid after client put medication in mouth.	____	____
d. Reminded client to lower chin while swallowing.	____	____
10. Closed containers.	____	____
11. Had client record medication(s) taken. (Aide recorded, if necessary.)	____	____
12. Stored materials in proper location.	____	____
13. Washed hands.	____	____
14. Recorded what was done. Reported any unusual conditions to supervisor.	____	____

Comments:

Evaluator's Signature: _____

Date: _____

PROCEDURE 18-2. ASSISTING WITH RECTAL SUPPOSITORIES

Name: _____

	S	UN
1. Explained procedure to client.	___	___
2. Checked care plan and medication sheet.	___	___
3. Washed hands.	___	___
4. Obtained necessary materials.	___	___
5. Provided privacy.	___	___
6. Assisted client into bed and into Sims' position.	___	___
7. Removed clothing to expose anal area.	___	___
8. Checked label on suppository for:	___	___
• Right drug	___	___
• Right client	___	___
• Right dose	___	___
• Right route	___	___
• Right time	___	___
9. Unwrapped suppository.	___	___
10. Applied water-soluble lubricant to suppository.	___	___
11. Gave glove to client to put on.	___	___
12. Handed suppository to client to insert into rectum. Guided client's hand, if necessary.	___	___
13. Observed as client inserted medication and wiped anus with toilet tissue.	___	___
14. Had client remove and discard glove into waste container.	___	___
15. Helped client to wash hands.	___	___
16. Discarded used materials in waste container.	___	___
17. Had client record medication(s) taken. (Aide recorded, if necessary.)	___	___
18. Reminded client to remain on side for 15 to 20 minutes to allow suppository to melt and medication to be absorbed.	___	___
19. Washed hands.	___	___
20. Recorded what was done. Reported any unusual conditions to supervisor.	___	___

Comments:

Evaluator's Signature: _____

Date: _____

PROCEDURE 18-3. ASSISTING WITH EYE MEDICATIONS OR OINTMENT

Name: _____

	S	UN
1. Explained procedure to client.	___	___
2. Checked care plan and medication sheet.	___	___
3. Washed hands. Put on disposable gloves (optional).	___	___
4. Obtained necessary materials.	___	___
5. Helped client to wash hands.	___	___
6. Checked label on prescription container for the following:	___	___
• Right drug: Made certain that preparation was for use in eyes only.	___	___
• Right client	___	___
• Right dose: Made certain the strength of the solution/ointment in the container was correct.	___	___
• Right route: Which eye, or both eyes.	___	___
• Right time	___	___
7. Loosened lid on container, if client was unable to do so.	___	___
8. Placed container within client's reach or handed to client as necessary. Made sure client was wearing eyeglasses, if needed.	___	___
9. Held mirror so client could see to administer eye medication.	___	___
10. Removed client's eyeglasses, if worn.	___	___
11. Assisted client with:	___	___

Eye Medications

	S	UN
a. Guided client's hand to grasp lower lid.	___	___
b. Observed that client looked up and released drops into lower lid.	___	___
c. Observed that client closed eye to distribute medication.	___	___
d. Made sure that dropper did not touch client's eye.	___	___

Eye Ointment

	S	UN
a. Guided client's hand to grasp lower eyelid.	___	___
b. Observed that client looked up and squeezed a small ribbon of ointment into the lower lid from inner corner of eye to outer corner of eye.	___	___
c. Observed that client closed eye to allow medication to melt and be distributed. Made sure that tip of tube did not touch eye surface	___	___
12. Resealed container.	___	___
13. Had client record medication(s) taken. (Aide recorded for client, if necessary.)	___	___
14. Stored materials in proper location.	___	___
15. Removed and discarded gloves (optional). Washed hands.	___	___
16. Recorded what was done. Reported any unusual conditions to supervisor.	___	___

Comments: _____

Evaluator's Signature: _____

Date: _____

PROCEDURE 18-4. ASSISTING WITH TRANSDERMAL DISKS OR PATCHES

Name: _____

	S	UN
1. Explained procedure to client.	___	___
2. Checked care plan and medication sheet.	___	___
3. Washed hands. Put on gloves (optional).	___	___
4. Obtained necessary materials.	___	___
5. Provided privacy.	___	___
6. Helped client to wash hands.	___	___
7. Checked label on container for the following:	___	___
• Right drug	___	___
• Right client	___	___
• Right dose	___	___
• Right route	___	___
• Right time	___	___
8. Had client remove and discard old disk or patch into waste container. Washed skin that had been covered by old disk or patch.	___	___
9. Asked client to select new site for new disk or patch (any area without hair), usually the chest or upper arm.	___	___
10. Observed as client applied new disk or patch to skin surface. Did not touch medicated surface with ungloved fingers.	___	___
11. Discarded wrapper and other used materials.	___	___
12. Had client record medication(s) taken. (Aide recorded for client, if necessary.)	___	___
13. Stored materials in proper location.	___	___
14. Removed and discarded gloves (optional). Washed hands.	___	___
15. Recorded what was done. Reported any unusual conditions to supervisor.	___	___

Comments:

Evaluator's Signature: _____

Date: _____

PROCEDURE 18-5. ASSISTING WITH MEDICATED GELS

Name: _____

	S	UN
1. Explained procedure to client.	___	___
2. Checked the care plan and medication sheet.	___	___
3. Washed hands.	___	___
4. Obtained necessary materials.	___	___
5. Provided privacy.	___	___
6. Helped client to wash hands.	___	___
7. Checked label on carton or tube for:	___	___
• Right drug	___	___
• Right client	___	___
• Right dose	___	___
• Right route	___	___
• Right time	___	___
8. Removed dosing card from package and placed on flat surface so client could read it.	___	___
9. Uncapped tube.	___	___
10. Observed as client applied gel onto dosing card.	___	___
11. Put cap back on tube.	___	___
12. Observed as client applied gel to prescribed area.	___	___
13. Helped client to wash hands (unless gel was applied to that area).	___	___
14. Had client record medication applied. (Aide recorded for client, if necessary.)	___	___
15. Rinsed and dried dosing card. Stored materials in proper location.	___	___
16. Washed hands.	___	___
17. Recorded what was done. Reported any unusual conditions to supervisor.	___	___

Comments:

Evaluator's Signature: _____

Date: _____

PROCEDURE 18-6. ASSISTING WITH METERED-DOSE INHALERS

Name: _____

	S	UN
1. Explained procedure to client.	___	___
2. Checked care plan and medication sheet.	___	___
3. Washed hands.	___	___
4. Obtained necessary materials.	___	___
5. Provided privacy.	___	___
6. Helped client to wash hands.	___	___
7. Checked label on prescription container for:	___	___
• Right drug	___	___
• Right client	___	___
• Right dose	___	___
• Right route	___	___
• Right time	___	___
8. Handed metered-dose inhaler to client, who then used it to inhale medication.	___	___
9. Had client record medication taken. (Aide recorded for client, if necessary.)	___	___
10. Cleaned inhaler, wearing disposable gloves, according to manufacturer's instructions. Stored in proper location.	___	___
11. Removed and discarded gloves. Washed hands.	___	___
12. Recorded what was done. Reported any unusual conditions to supervisor.	___	___
13. Assisted client with oral hygiene, as needed.	___	___

Comments:

Evaluator's Signature: _____

Date: _____

PROCEDURE 18-7. APPLYING A HOT WATER BAG

Name: _____

	S	UN
1. Explained procedure to client.	___	___
2. Washed hands.	___	___
3. Obtained necessary materials.	___	___
4. Provided privacy.	___	___
5. Filled hot water bag with water. Secured with stopper. Turned bag upside down to check for leaks.	___	___
6. Removed stopper and emptied bag.	___	___
7. Ran more hot water and tested with cooking thermometer. Adjusted water temperature to 115° to 130° F or 46° to 54.4° C.	___	___
8. Filled bag one-third to one-half full.	___	___
9. Laid bag flat to remove air. Placed stopper in bag while it was still flat.	___	___
10. Covered bag with soft cloth or towel. Applied bag to client's affected area.	___	___
11. Wrote on paper the time the bag was applied.	___	___
12. Refilled bag when it became cool.	___	___
13. Checked client's skin every 10 minutes for danger signs.	___	___
14. Removed bag according to time required. Wrote time of removal on paper.	___	___
15. Removed stopper, emptied bag, and hung bag upside down to dry. Placed cloth or towel in laundry container.	___	___
16. Washed hands.	___	___
17. Recorded what was done. Reported any unusual conditions to supervisor.	___	___
18. When bag was dry, blew air into it, and replaced stopper to prevent inside of bag from sticking together. Stored in proper location.	___	___

Comments:

Evaluator's Signature: _____

Date: _____

PROCEDURE 18-8. APPLYING A HOT OR COLD PACK

Name: _____

		S	UN
1.	Explained procedure to client.	____	____
2.	Washed hands.	____	____
3.	Obtained necessary materials.	____	____
4.	Provided privacy.	____	____
5.	Placed hot pack in microwave and heated according to manufacturer's directions or removed cold pack from freezer.	____	____
6.	Covered pack with soft cloth, towel, or cover and applied to client's affected area.	____	____
7.	Wrote on paper the time the pack was applied.	____	____
8.	Checked client's skin every 10 minutes for danger signs.	____	____
9.	Removed pack according to time required. Wrote time of removal on paper.	____	____
10.	Stored pack according to manufacturer's directions. Placed cloth, towel, or cover in laundry container.	____	____
11.	Washed hands.	____	____
12.	Recorded what was done. Reported any unusual conditions to supervisor.	____	____

Comments:

Evaluator's Signature: _____

Date: _____

PROCEDURE 18-9. APPLYING HOT COMPRESSES

Name: _____

	S	UN
1. Explained procedure to client.	____	____
2. Washed hands.	____	____
3. Obtained necessary materials.	____	____
4. Provided privacy.	____	____
5. Placed waterproof protector pad under the body part where compress was to be applied.	____	____
6. Filled basin or container one-half to two-thirds full of water at 105° to 115° F (40.5° to 46.1° C). Checked temperature with cooking thermometer.	____	____
7. Put on gloves.	____	____
8. Placed compress in the water.	____	____
9. Wrung out compress and applied to area. Noted time applied.	____	____
10. Covered compress quickly with plastic wrap. Secured edges of plastic wrap with tape. Covered with bath towel.	____	____
11. Wrote on paper the time compress was applied.	____	____
12. Applied, according to instructions, hot water bag or rubber-protected heating pad over plastic wrap to keep compress hot.	____	____
13. Checked client's skin every 10 minutes for danger signs.	____	____
14. Changed compress if cooling occurred.	____	____
15. Removed compress according to time required.	____	____
16. Wrote time of removal on paper.	____	____
17. Patted area dry with towel. Discarded used compress. Placed used cloths or towels in laundry container.	____	____
18. Removed and discarded gloves.	____	____
19. Washed hands.	____	____
20. Cleaned and stored materials in proper location.	____	____
21. Recorded what was done. Reported any unusual conditions to supervisor.	____	____

Comments:

Evaluator's Signature: _____

Date: _____

PROCEDURE 18-10. APPLYING HOT SOAKS

Name: _____

	S	UN
1. Explained procedure to client.	___	___
2. Washed hands.	___	___
3. Obtained necessary materials.	___	___
4. Provided privacy.	___	___
5. Assisted client to comfortable position.	___	___
6. Placed waterproof protector pad under the area to be soaked.	___	___
7. Filled basin or container one-half full of water 105° to 110 °F (40.5° to 43.3° C). Checked temperature with cooking thermometer.	___	___
8. Exposed only the part to be soaked.	___	___
9. Placed area to be soaked into water.	___	___
10. Checked water temperature and skin of area being soaked every 10 minutes. Removed body part from water if danger signs were noticed.	___	___
11. Removed body part from water according to time required.	___	___
12. Wrote time of removal on paper.	___	___
13. Patted body part dry. Assisted client to replace clothing and to get comfortable.	___	___
14. Cleaned and stored materials in proper location.	___	___
15. Put used towel in laundry container.	___	___
16. Washed hands.	___	___
17. Recorded what was done. Reported any unusual conditions to supervisor.	___	___

Comments:

Evaluator's Signature: _____

Date: _____

PROCEDURE 18-11. GIVING A SITZ BATH

Name: _____

	S	UN
1. Explained procedure to client.	___	___
2. Washed hands.	___	___
3. Obtained necessary materials.	___	___
4. Assisted client to bathroom or commode.	___	___
5. Provided privacy.	___	___
6. Put on gloves.	___	___
7. Helped client to remove clothing from below waist.	___	___
8. Asked client to remove and discard dressing or pad, if worn. Assisted, if needed. Observed amount and color of drainage.	___	___
9. Asked client to void before beginning the procedure.	___	___
10. Raised toilet seat. Placed sitz bowl so that drainage holes were at the back of the toilet. Filled half of plastic sitz bowl with warm water, 94° to 98° F (34° to 37° C). Checked temperature with cooking thermometer.	___	___
11. Closed side clamp of bag tubing. Filled water bag with warm water, 120° F (49° C). Hung bag so that it was higher than the toilet (on towel bar, top of toilet tank, or vanity).	___	___
12. Assisted client to sit in sitz bowl. If client felt cold, covered shoulders and knees with blanket or towel.	___	___
13. Placed tube end of water bag in outlet at front of the bowl.	___	___
14. Instructed client to open clamp of water bag to let warmer water into the bowl when water began to cool. Assisted as needed.	___	___
15. Instructed client to call for assistance, if needed. Explained that the procedure will take 15 to 20 minutes.	___	___
16. Removed and discarded gloves.	___	___
17. Washed hands.	___	___
18. Checked client's condition every 5 minutes or more frequently, if needed.	___	___
19. When time was up, clamped tubing and removed from sitz bath.	___	___
20. Washed hands. Put on second pair of gloves.	___	___
21. Assisted client to slowly assume standing position.	___	___
22. Inspected perineal area, and noted any drainage in water. Dried area and reapplied dressing or pad, if needed.	___	___
23. Assisted client to dress, as needed, and returned to bed or chair.	___	___
24. Emptied and disinfected plastic bowl. Flushed tubing with warm water and cleaned end of tubing. Returned equipment to proper location.	___	___
25. Removed and discarded gloves.	___	___
26. Washed hands.	___	___
27. Straightened bathroom.	___	___
28. Recorded on care record. Noted color and amount of drainage on dressing or pad. Reported any unusual conditions to supervisor.	___	___

Comments: _____

Evaluator's Signature: _____

Date: _____

PROCEDURE 18-12. APPLYING AN ICE BAG

Name: _____

	S	UN
1. Explained procedure to client.	___	___
2. Washed hands.	___	___
3. Obtained necessary materials.	___	___
4. Provided privacy.	___	___
5. Filled ice bag with water. Secured with stopper. Turned bag upside down to check for leaks.	___	___
6. Removed stopper and emptied bag.	___	___
7. Crushed the ice and filled bag one-half to two-thirds full.	___	___
8. Laid bag flat to remove air. Placed stopper in bag while it was still flat.	___	___
9. Covered bag with soft cloth or towel and applied to client's affected area.	___	___
10. Wrote on paper the time bag was applied.	___	___
11. Added ice as bag warmed. Changed towel if it became moist.	___	___
12. Checked client's skin every 10 minutes for danger signs.	___	___
13. Removed bag according to time required. Wrote time of removal on paper.	___	___
14. Removed stopper, emptied bag, and placed bag upside down to dry. Placed cloth or towel in laundry container to be washed.	___	___
15. Washed hands.	___	___
16. Recorded what was done. Reported any unusual conditions to supervisor.	___	___
17. When bag was dry, blew air into it, and replaced stopper to prevent insides of bag from sticking together. Stored in proper location.	___	___

Comments:

Evaluator's Signature: _____

Date: _____

PROCEDURE 18-13. APPLYING COLD COMPRESSES

Name: _____

	S	**UN**
1. Explained procedure to client.	——	——
2. Washed hands.	——	——
3. Obtained necessary materials.	——	——
4. Provided privacy.	——	——
5. Placed waterproof protector pad under the body part where compress was to be applied.	——	——
6. Filled basin or container one-half to two-thirds full with ice water.	——	——
7. Put on gloves.	——	——
8. Placed compress in water.	——	——
9. Wrung out compress and applied to area.	——	——
10. Covered compress quickly with plastic wrap. Secured edges of plastic wrap with tape. Covered with bath towel.	——	——
11. Wrote on paper the time compress was applied.	——	——
12. Checked client's skin every 10 minutes for danger signs.	——	——
13. Changed compress when warming occurred.	——	——
14. Removed compress according to time required.	——	——
15. Wrote time of removal on paper.	——	——
16. Patted area dry with towel. Discarded used gauze squares or compresses. Placed used washcloths and towels in laundry container.	——	——
17. Removed and discarded gloves.	——	——
18. Washed hands.	——	——
19. Cleaned and stored materials in proper location.	——	——
20. Recorded what was done. Reported any unusual conditions to supervisor.	——	——

Comments:

Evaluator's Signature: _____

Date: _____

PROCEDURE 18-14. REMOVING A SOILED DRESSING AND APPLYING A CLEAN, DRY DRESSING

Name: _____

	S	UN
1. Explained procedure to client.	___	___
2. Washed hands.	___	___
3. Obtained necessary materials.	___	___
4. Provided privacy.	___	___
5. Cut lengths of tape needed and hung them on edge of table for later use.	___	___
6. Put on gloves.	___	___

Removing Soiled Dressing

	S	UN
7. Exposed area where dressing was to be removed.	___	___
8. Placed paper or plastic bag nearby.	___	___
9. Removed all tape from the skin by pulling tape toward dressing/wound.	___	___
10. Gently removed soiled dressing using tongs or clothespin to grasp edges. If tongs or clothespin were not available, grasped the cleanest part of the dressing and removed. Inspected dressing and skin. Noted color, amount of drainage, and odor. Discarded into paper bag.	___	___
11. Discarded soiled gloves. Washed hands. Put on clean gloves.	___	___

Applying Clean, Dry Dressing

	S	UN
12. Removed clean, dry dressing from cover, touching edge of dressing only.	___	___
13. Applied dressing to area.	___	___
14. Took strips of precut tape and applied to secure dressing.	___	___
15. Placed dressing cover in paper bag and discarded.	___	___
16. Removed and discarded gloves in paper or plastic bag.	___	___
17. Washed hands.	___	___
18. Recorded what was done. Reported any unusual conditions to supervisor.	___	___

Comments:

Evaluator's Signature: _____

Date: _____

PROCEDURE 18-15. APPLYING ELASTIC STOCKINGS

Name: _____

	S	UN
1. Explained procedure to client.	____	____
2. Washed hands.	____	____
3. Obtained elastic stockings.	____	____
4. Provided privacy.	____	____
5. Placed client in supine position.	____	____
6. Exposed legs. Checked to see that legs were clean and dry.	____	____
7. Turned stocking inside out by placing one hand into sock, holding toe of sock with other hand, and pulling.	____	____
8. Placed client's toes into foot of stocking. Made sure sock was smooth.	____	____
9. Slid remaining portion of sock over client's foot and heel. Made sure foot fit into toe and heel positions of sock. (Sock is now right side out.)	____	____
10. Pulled stocking up over client's calf until stocking was fully extended.	____	____
11. Inspected stocking to make sure that there were no wrinkles or binding at top of stocking.	____	____
12. Made sure client was safe and comfortable.	____	____
13. Washed hands.	____	____
14. Recorded what was done. Reported any unusual conditions to supervisor.	____	____
15. Checked circulation regularly according to care plan.	____	____

Comments:

Evaluator's Signature: _____

Date: _____

PROCEDURE 18-16. APPLYING ELASTIC BANDAGES

Name: _____

	S	UN
1. Explained procedure to client.	___	___
2. Washed hands.	___	___
3. Obtained necessary materials.	___	___
4. Provided privacy.	___	___
5. Assisted client to comfortable position: supine for legs and feet; other positions according to care plan and part to be bandaged.	___	___
6. Exposed part. Checked to see that it was clean and dry.	___	___
7. Held bandage with roll up.	___	___
8. Applied one end of bandage to smallest part (e.g., wrist, ankle).	___	___
9. Wrapped two turns to anchor bandage.	___	___
10. Continued wrapping in spiral turns upward (overlapped previous turn by two thirds). Applied firmly but NOT TOO TIGHTLY.	___	___
11. Fastened end with clip, pin, or tape.	___	___
12. Washed hands.	___	___
13. Recorded what was done. Reported any unusual conditions to supervisor.	___	___
14. Checked for proper circulation regularly according to care plan.	___	___

Comments:

Evaluator's Signature: _____

Date: _____

PROCEDURE 20-1. BATHING AN INFANT: SPONGE BATH

Name: _____

	S	UN
1. Washed hands.	___	___
2. Obtained necessary materials.	___	___
3. Placed all materials within easy reach. Spread hooded towel or receiving blanket on flat surface near where baby would be bathed.	___	___
4. Placed baby on receiving blanket or hooded towel next to basin of warm water. Always kept one hand on baby. Never left baby unattended.	___	___
5. Began with baby's head:	___	___
a. Wet a cotton ball with plain water and gently cleaned eye by wiping from inner corner to outer corner. Discarded cotton ball. Used new one to clean other eye.	___	___
b. Wet washcloth and sponged face, ears, and folds in neck. Patted dry.	___	___
c. Picked up baby, holding in the football hold, facing upright. Held head over basin. With free hand, wet washcloth, and wrung it out over baby's scalp. Put small amount of soap on palm of hand, and rubbed it gently onto baby's scalp. Rinsed by wringing wet washcloth over baby's head. Dried gently. Covered head with hooded towel or receiving blanket.	___	___
6. Removed shirt. Washed chest, upper abdomen, arms, and hands. Patted dry. Turned baby, washed and dried back.	___	___
7. Put clean shirt on baby.	___	___
8. Cleaned umbilical cord area with alcohol (according to care plan).	___	___
9. Removed lower clothing. Washed and dried legs and feet.	___	___
10. Put on gloves.	___	___
11. Removed diaper. Wiped any feces away with tissue, and cleaned perineal area. Discarded diaper or set aside for laundry. Washed perineum:	___	___
a. For girl: washed from front to back, rinsed thoroughly, and gently patted dry.	___	___
b. For boy: washed entire scrotum and cared for circumcision according to care plan.	___	___
12. Put dry diaper on baby.	___	___
13. Removed and discarded gloves.	___	___
14. Finished dressing baby. Wrapped baby in receiving blanket.	___	___
15. Placed baby in a safe and comfortable position.	___	___
16. Cleaned materials and returned to proper location.	___	___
17. Recorded what was done. Reported any unusual observations to supervisor.	___	___

Comments:

Evaluator's Signature: _____

Date: _____

PROCEDURE 20-2. BATHING AN INFANT: TUB BATH

Name: _____

	S	UN
1. Washed hands.	___	___
2. Obtained necessary materials.	___	___
3. Placed all materials within easy reach. Spread hooded towel or receiving blanket on flat surface near where baby will be bathed.	___	___
4. Placed baby on receiving blanket or hooded towel next to basin of warm water. Always kept one hand on baby. Never left baby unattended.	___	___
5. Began with the head:	___	___
a. Wet a cotton ball with plain water and gently cleaned eye by wiping from inner corner to outer corner. Discarded cotton ball. Used new one to clean baby's other eye.	___	___
b. Wet washcloth and sponged face, ears, and folds in neck. Patted dry.	___	___
c. Picked up baby, holding in the football hold, facing upright. Held baby's head over basin. With free hand, wet washcloth, and wrung it out over baby's scalp. Put small amount of soap on palm of hand, and rubbed it gently onto baby's scalp. Rinsed by wringing wet washcloth over baby's head. Dried gently. Covered head with hooded towel or receiving blanket.	___	___
6. Laid baby back on flat surface.	___	___
7. Removed shirt.	___	___
8. Put on gloves.	___	___
9. Removed diaper. Wiped any feces away with tissue, and cleaned perineal area. Discarded diaper or set aside for laundry.	___	___
10. Removed and discarded gloves.	___	___
11. Held infant:	___	___
a. Placed left hand under baby's shoulders. Thumb over the left shoulder. Aide's hand held the upper left arm.	___	___
b. Used right hand to support baby's buttocks. Slid hand under baby's thigh. Held baby's left thigh with right hand.	___	___
12. Lowered baby into water feet first.	___	___
13. Washed front of infant's body using right hand.	___	___
14. Changed hold:	___	___
a. Used right hand to support baby in a sitting forward position.	___	___
b. Supported and held fingers around baby's upper arm and placed hand under infant's chin, as in a lap position for burping.	___	___
15. Washed baby's back.	___	___
16. Returned to previous position.	___	___
17. Washed genital area.	___	___

18. Lifted baby out of water and onto towel. ___ ___

19. Wrapped baby in towel and covered his or her head. ___ ___

20. Patted baby dry. ___ ___

21. Put dry diaper on baby. ___ ___

22. Finished dressing baby. Wrapped baby in receiving blanket. ___ ___

23. Placed baby in safe and comfortable position. ___ ___

24. Cleaned materials and returned to proper location. ___ ___

25. Recorded what was done. Reported any unusual observations to supervisor. ___ ___

Comments:

Evaluator's Signature: _____

Date: _____

PROCEDURE 20-3. DRESSING AN INFANT

Name: _____

	S	UN
1. Applied shirt:	___	___
a. Stretched neck of shirt and pulled over baby's head.	___	___
b. Placed hand inside sleeve, reached up through sleeve to grasp baby's hand, and pulled through.	___	___
c. Repeated on other side.	___	___
d. Pulled shirt down over chest. If umbilical stump present, folded bottom of shirt up to avoid rubbing.	___	___
2. Applied one-piece sleeper:	___	___
a. Unfastened all snaps on sleeper.	___	___
b. Laid garment on flat surface.	___	___
c. Placed baby on garment.	___	___
d. Inserted feet into lower portion of sleeper.	___	___
e. Reached through sleeves (as for shirt) to put on upper portion of sleeper.	___	___
f. Snapped up garment.	___	___
3. Applied booties:	___	___
a. Rolled bootie over hand, inside out.	___	___
b. Grasped infant's toes and turned bootie up and over foot with other hand.	___	___

Comments:

Evaluator's Signature: _____

Date: _____

PROCEDURE 20-4. CHANGING A DIAPER

Name: _____

	S	UN
1. Washed hands.	___	___
2. Obtained necessary materials	___	___
3. Put on gloves.	___	___
4. Placed baby on changing surface near materials. Made sure to protect baby from rolling off of surface.	___	___
5. Opened soiled diaper.	___	___
6. Wiped genital area with front of diaper, if dry. Wiped from front to back.	___	___
7. Rolled diaper so that urine and feces were inside. Set aside for later disposal.	___	___
8. Washed the perineal area with soap and water or used baby wipes. Rinsed and dried thoroughly.	___	___
9. Provided cord and circumcision care according to care plan.	___	___
10. Raised baby's legs. Placed clean diaper in place. Folded cloth diaper to better fit baby, if needed:	___	___
a. For girl, extra fold in back.	___	___
b. For boy, extra fold in front.	___	___
11. Pinned or fastened diaper in place. Kept diaper below umbilical stump. Was careful not to stick baby with diaper pin. Had finger under diaper when pin was inserted.	___	___
12. Applied plastic pants (if cloth diaper used).	___	___
13. Placed baby in safe and comfortable position.	___	___
14. Rinsed or dumped feces from diaper into toilet. Flushed toilet. Rinsed cloth diaper with cool water and placed in diaper pail for laundering. Discarded disposable diaper in garbage.	___	___
15. Removed and discarded gloves.	___	___
16. Washed hands.	___	___
17. Recorded what was done. Reported any unusual observations to supervisor.	___	___

Comments:

Evaluator's Signature: _____

Date: _____

PROCEDURE 20-5. ASSISTING MOTHER TO BREAST-FEED

Name: _____

	S	UN
1. Washed hands.	___	___
2. Had mother wash her hands. Nipples were washed with plain water (if called for in care plan) in a circular motion from nipple outward.	___	___
3. Helped mother to a comfortable position.	___	___
a. In chair with feet up on a stool.	___	___
b. In bed with pillows behind back and head for support; adjusted pillows until mother was comfortable.	___	___
4. Changed baby's diaper, if needed.	___	___
5. Brought baby to mother.	___	___
6. Had mother touch infant's cheek on side nearest the breast.	___	___
7. Observed that mother held back breast tissue so baby could "latch on" to entire nipple and most of areola. Infant's lips covered this area. Baby's tongue was under nipple.	___	___
8. Observed that baby nursed for about 10 minutes on each breast. If baby fell asleep during feeding, mother removed baby from breast; awakened baby by washing face, changing diaper, or tapping feet; put baby back to breast.	___	___
9. Reminded mother how to remove baby from breast: by inserting her finger into corner of baby's mouth to break the suction.	___	___
10. Observed that mother burped baby before moving baby to other breast.	___	___
11. When feeding was over, changed diaper.	___	___
12. Placed baby on back.	___	___
13. Observed that mother massaged a little milk or colostrum onto nipples after feeding, if desired. Breasts were air dried. Nipples were kept dry.	___	___
14. Assisted mother with dressing, if necessary. A nursing bra was worn, if desired.	___	___
15. Recorded what was done. Reported any unusual findings to supervisor.	___	___

Comments:

Evaluator's Signature: _____

Date: _____

PROCEDURE 20-6. PREPARING FORMULA FROM POWDER

Name: _____

	S	UN
1. Washed hands.	___	___
2. Obtained necessary materials.	___	___
3. Boiled water and allowed it to cool.	___	___
4. Poured cooled water into bottle.	___	___
5. Added powdered formula using scoop, according to label instructions.	___	___
6. Shook well to mix.	___	___
7. Capped, sealed, and stored bottles in refrigerator until needed.	___	___

Comments:

Evaluator's Signature: _____

Date: _____

PROCEDURE 20-7. PREPARING FORMULA USING CONCENTRATED FORMULA

Name: _____

	S	UN
1. Washed hands.	___	___
2. Obtained necessary materials.	___	___
3. Boiled water and allowed it to cool.	___	___
4. Washed can lid with hot, soapy water. Rinsed lid and opened can.	___	___
5. Poured appropriate amount of water into bottle.	___	___
6. Added appropriate amount of formula through funnel into bottle.	___	___
7. Shook well to mix.	___	___
8. Capped, sealed, and stored formula in refrigerator until needed.	___	___

Comments:

Evaluator's Signature: _____

Date: _____

PROCEDURE 20-8. PREPARING FORMULA FROM READY-TO-USE SUPPLY

Name: _____

	S	UN
1. Washed hands.	____	____
2. Obtained necessary materials.	____	____
3. Washed off can lid with hot, soapy water. Rinsed lid and opened can.	____	____
4. Poured formula into bottle using funnel.	____	____
5. Capped, sealed, and stored bottles in refrigerator until needed.	____	____

Comments:

Evaluator's Signature: _____

Date: _____

PROCEDURE 20-9. ASSISTING MOTHER TO BOTTLE-FEED

Name: _____

	S	UN
1. Washed hands.	___	___
2. Obtained necessary materials.	___	___
3. Warmed bottle (if cold) by placing in a pan of warm water until bottle was about room temperature.	___	___
4. Had mother wash her hands.	___	___
5. Helped mother to a comfortable position.	___	___
6. Changed baby's diaper, if necessary.	___	___
7. Brought bottle and baby to mother.	___	___
8. Bottle was tilted so that neck of bottle and nipple were always covered with formula. Did not prop bottle.	___	___
9. Had mother burp baby halfway through feeding and at end.	___	___
10. Feeding was discontinued when baby was no longer eating.	___	___
11. Changed diaper.	___	___
12. Placed baby on back.	___	___
13. Washed hands.	___	___
14. Recorded what was done and the amount of formula taken. Reported any unusual observations to supervisor.	___	___

Comments:

Evaluator's Signature: _____

Date: _____

PROCEDURE 22-1. ASSISTING POSTOPERATIVE CLIENTS TO DEEP BREATHE AND COUGH

Name: _____

	S	UN
Deep Breathing		
1. Explained procedure to client.	____	____
2. Provided privacy	____	____
3. Assisted client into sitting position.	____	____
4. Had client place hands over lower end of rib cage, with tips of middle fingers just touching each other.	____	____
5. Instructed client to deep breathe by:	____	____
a. Exhaling until the ribs move down as far as possible	____	____
b. Breathing in through the nose as deeply as possible (Client should be able to feel fingers separate during inhalation.)	____	____
c. Holding the breath for a count of "3"	____	____
d. Exhaling slowly through pursed lips until the ribs move as far down as possible	____	____
6. Repeated procedure according to care plan (usually every 1 to 2 hours while client was awake).	____	____
7. Recorded what was done. Reported any unusual observations to supervisor.	____	____
Coughing		
1. Explained procedure to client.	____	____
2. Asked client to place interlaced fingers or small pillow over incision.	____	____
3. Had client take two deep breaths.	____	____
4. Told client to take another deep breath, hold for a count of "3," and then cough twice with mouth open. Did not let client cough on aide.	____	____
5. Repeated procedure according to care plan (usually two or three coughs per hour).	____	____
6. Recorded what was done. Reported any unusual observations to supervisor.	____	____

Comments:

Evaluator's Signature: _____

Date: _____

Skills Competency Checklists Record

Name: _____

Procedure	Date Taught	Date Successfully Demonstrated
10-1. Feeding the Client	_____	_____
11-1. Handwashing	_____	_____
11-2. Applying Gloves and Removing Contaminated Gloves	_____	_____
11-3. Disinfecting Using Wet Heat	_____	_____
11-4. Disinfecting Using Dry Heat	_____	_____
11-5. Making Bleach Solution	_____	_____
11-6. Making Vinegar Solution	_____	_____
11-7. Disinfecting With Household Solutions	_____	_____
11-8. Applying a Mask and Removing a Contaminated Mask	_____	_____
11-9. Applying a Gown and Removing a Contaminated Gown	_____	_____
11-10. Double Bagging	_____	_____
12-1. Raising Client's Head and Shoulders	_____	_____
12-2. Moving Client to the Side of the Bed	_____	_____
12-3. Moving Up in Bed When Client Can Help	_____	_____
12-4. Moving Up in Bed When Client Cannot Help	_____	_____
12-5. Positioning Client in the Supine (Back-Lying) Position	_____	_____
12-6. Positioning Client in the Fowler's (Semi-Sitting) Position	_____	_____
12-7. Positioning Client in the Lateral (Side-Lying) Position	_____	_____
12-8. Positioning Client in the Sims' Position	_____	_____
12-9. Positioning Client in the Prone (Abdominal) Position	_____	_____
12-10. Assisting Client to Sit on the Side of the Bed	_____	_____
12-11. Transferring Client From Bed to Chair/Wheelchair: Standing Transfer	_____	_____
12-12. Transferring Client From Bed to Chair/Wheelchair: Standing Transfer Using Transfer Belt	_____	_____
12-13. Returning Client to Bed	_____	_____
12-14. Applying a Transfer (Gait) Belt	_____	_____
12-15. Using a Mechanical Lift	_____	_____
13-1. Making a Closed Bed	_____	_____
13-2. Making an Open Bed	_____	_____

13-3. Making an Occupied Bed   _____ _____

13-4. Making a Mitered Corner   _____ _____

14-1. Brushing Teeth   _____ _____

14-2. Flossing Teeth   _____ _____

14-3. Mouth Care for the Unconscious Client   _____ _____

14-4. Caring for Dentures   _____ _____

14-5. Giving a Complete Bed Bath   _____ _____

14-6. Giving a Tub Bath   _____ _____

14-7. Giving a Back Rub   _____ _____

14-8. Giving Perineal Care   _____ _____

14-9. Caring for Nails and Feet   _____ _____

14-10. Assisting Client With Hair Care   _____ _____

14-11. Giving a Shampoo   _____ _____

14-12. Shaving the Male Client   _____ _____

14-13. Helping Client to Dress   _____ _____

14-14. Helping Client With an Intravenous (IV) Line to Remove Used
       Clothing and Apply Clean Clothing   _____ _____

14-15. Helping With Range-of-Motion Exercises in Bed: General Procedure _____ _____

15-1. Giving and Removing a Bedpan   _____ _____

15-2. Giving and Removing a Urinal   _____ _____

15-3. Measuring and Recording Intake and Output   _____ _____

15-4. Care of the Client With an Indwelling Catheter   _____ _____

15-5. Emptying a Catheter Drainage Bag   _____ _____

15-6. Applying a Condom Catheter   _____ _____

16-1. Collecting a Routine Urine Specimen   _____ _____

16-2. Collecting a "Clean Catch" or Midstream Urine Specimen _____ _____

16-3. Collecting a 24-Hour Urine Specimen   _____ _____

16-4. Straining Urine   _____ _____

16-5. Collecting a Stool Specimen   _____ _____

16-6. Collecting a Sputum Specimen   _____ _____

17-1. Cleaning a Thermometer   _____ _____

17-2. Taking an Oral Temperature (With a Regular Thermometer) _____ _____

17-3. Taking an Oral Temperature (With an Electronic Thermometer) _____ _____

17-4. Taking an Oral Temperature (With a Single-Use Thermometer) _____ _____

17-5. Taking an Axillary Temperature   _____ _____

17-6. Taking a Temperature Using a Tympanic Thermometer   _____ _____

17-7. Taking a Rectal Temperature _____ _____

17-8. Taking a Radial Pulse _____ _____

17-9. Taking Respirations _____ _____

17-10. Measuring Blood Pressure _____ _____

18-1. Assisting With Oral Medications _____ _____

18-2. Assisting With Rectal Suppositories _____ _____

18-3. Assisting With Eye Medications or Ointment _____ _____

18-4. Assisting With Transdermal Disks or Patches _____ _____

18-5. Assisting With Medicated Gels _____ _____

18-6. Assisting With Metered-Dose Inhalers _____ _____

18-7. Applying a Hot Water Bag _____ _____

18-8. Applying a Hot or Cold Pack _____ _____

18-9. Applying Hot Compresses _____ _____

18-10. Applying Hot Soaks _____ _____

18-11. Giving a Sitz Bath _____ _____

18-12. Applying an Ice Bag _____ _____

18-13. Applying Cold Compresses _____ _____

18-14. Removing a Soiled Dressing and Applying a Clean, Dry Dressing _____ _____

18-15. Applying Elastic Stockings _____ _____

18-16. Applying Elastic Bandages _____ _____

20-1. Bathing an Infant: Sponge Bath _____ _____

20-2. Bathing an Infant: Tub Bath _____ _____

20-3. Dressing an Infant _____ _____

20-4. Changing a Diaper _____ _____

20-5. Assisting Mother to Breast-Feed _____ _____

20-6. Preparing Formula From Powder _____ _____

20-7. Preparing Formula Using Concentrated Formula _____ _____

20-8. Preparing Formula From Ready-to-Use Supply _____ _____

20-9. Assisting Mother to Bottle-Feed _____ _____

22-1. Assisting Postoperative Clients to Deep Breathe and Cough _____ _____

Instructor's Name: _____